KU-685-097

Healthcare Reform and Poverty in Latin America

Edited by

Peter Lloyd-Sherlock

Institute of Latin American Studies
31 Tavistock Square, London WC1H 9HA
http://www.sas.ac.uk/ilas/publicat.htm

UNIVERSITY OF HERTFORDSHIRE
HATFIELD CAMPUS LRC
HATFIELD AL10 9AD 351727

BIB
1900039346

CLASS
362.1098 HER

LOCATION
FWL

BARCODE
4404633427

Institute of Latin American Studies
School of Advanced Study
University of London

British Library Cataloguing-in-Publication Data
   A catalogue record for this book is available
   from the British Library

ISBN   1 900039 34 6

©Institute of Latin American Studies
   University of London, 2000

Printed and bound by Short Run Press Limited Exeter

CONTENTS

Notes on Contributors

Christopher Abel is Senior Lecturer in Latin American History at University College London and an Associate Fellow of the Institute of Latin American Studies, University of London. He is currently completing a monograph on the history of healthcare in Colombia during the coffee ascendancy, 1910s to 1970s, and is co-organiser (LSE and ILAS) of a forthcoming (2001) EU-funded conference on 'Exclusion and Engagement: Social Policy in Latin America' for publication by ILAS, London, with Dr Colin M. Lewis, with whom he co-edited the book *Welfare, Poverty and Development in Latin America*, published by Macmillan in 1994.

Sarah Atkinson is a Senior Lecturer at the University of Manchester, School of Geography. Her research includes the social and political contexts of the implementation of policy within health systems, aspects of urban health policy and the role of values and norms on practice within health systems and has been working most recently in Zambia, Brazil and Chile.

Armando Barrientos is Principal Lecturer in Economics at the University of Hertfordshire. His recent publications include 'Pension Reform in Latin America' (1998) published by Ashgate, 'Work, Retirement and Vulnerability of Older Persons in Latin America. What are the Lessons for Pension Design?', in *Journal of International Development* (2000) and 'Reforming Health Insurance in Argentina and Chile', in *Health Policy and Planning* (2000), with Peter Lloyd-Sherlock.

Julio Frenk is Executive Director, Evidence and Information for Policy of the World Health Organisation, Executive Vice President of the Mexican Health Foundation and Director of the Center for Health and the Economy, Mexico. Over the years he has held several lectureships and professorships at the University of Michigan, the School of Public Health of Mexico, the National Autonomous University of Mexico, the National Institute of Public Health, Harvard University and the Iberoamerican University. In addition, he has served as advisor to the Technical Department for Latin America and the Caribbean at the World Bank.

Octavio Gómez-Dantés is Director of Health Policy and Planning at the Center for Health Systems Research of the National Institute of Public Health, Mexico. His research areas are health policies and international health. Recent publications include: Daniels, N., Bryant J., Castaño R.A., Gómez-Dantés O. and Pannarunothai, K., 'Benchmarks of Fairness for Health Care Reform', *WHO Bulletin*, vol. 78, no. 6, pp. 740–50 and Gómez-Dantes, O., 'La regulación de la práctica médica en México', *Investigación Clínica*, vol. 51, no. 4, pp. 245-53.

Richard M. Garfield is a nurse, epidemiologist and Professor at Columbia University. Since 1980 he has measured the impact of wars and humanitarian crises on civilian populations. His current research includes: identification of long term trends in casualties among civilians in wars and complex humanitarian emergencies; the impact of economic embargoes on health and well-being of civilians, with detailed case studies in Iraq, Haiti and Cuba; the impact of structural adjustment programmes on the services in developing countries; and assessment of the value and limitations of the Oil for Food Programme in Iraq

Timothy H. Holtz at the time of writing his chapter was Assistant Clinical Professor in the Department of Family Medicine of the Boston University School of

Medicine. He is currently based in Atlanta as a physician and officer for the Centers for Disease Control and Prevention.

Núria Homedes is Associate Professor at the School of Public Health, University of Texas at Houston. Previously, she worked for the Rural Health Office at the University of Arizona and the World Bank. She is a co-editor of *Farmacos*, an electronic journal dedicated to fostering the adequate use of pharmaceuticals. She is currently studying health reform in Latin America.

Peter Lloyd-Sherlock is Lecturer in Social Development in the School of Development Studies at the University of East Anglia. He works on Social Policy in Developing Countries, concentrating on Latin America, particularly Argentina and Brazil. He is author of *Old Age and Urban Poverty in the Developing World* (Basingstoke: Macmillan, 1997).

Juan Luis Londoño is former Minister of Health of Colombia. He is Senior Economist at the Office of the Chief Economist, Inter-American Development Bank, Washington, DC. When his chapter was written, he was Principal Human Resource Economist, Technical Department for Latin and the Caribbean, The World Bank, Washington, DC. He is editor of the magazine *Dinero*.

Ana Carolina Paz-Narváez is Professor in the Department of Public Health (Universidad Centroamericana José Simeón Cañas UCA, San Salvador). Before joining UCA, she headed the Community Health Unit of the National University of El Salvador and coordinated health promoters programmes. Her field of interest includes community organisation and health.

Ernesto A. Selva-Sutter is the Head of the Department of Public Health at the Universidad Centroamericana José Simeón Cañas UCA, San Salvador. Previously he was the Acting President of the Universidad Nacional de El Salvador and Associate Dean at the same university. His field of interest is the social and structural dimensions of health and illness.

Olga Solas is a sociologist and teaches at the Escuela Andaluza de Salud Pública (Granada, Spain). She has been a consultant with the Inter-American Development Bank, the European Union, World Bank and the Ibero-American Cooperation Agency. Her field of interest includes health policies and reform, health and migration and human resources management.

Antonio Ugalde teaches sociology at the University of Texas-Austin. He is a co-editor of the electronic journal *Farmacos* and member of the advisory board of *Social Science and Medicine* and of *Cuadernos Médico Sociales* (Argentina). His field of interest is health policy, social change and North-South relations.

Francisco José Yepes Lujan is a doctor and surgeon, formerly Executive Director of the Colombian Health Association (ASSALUD) he is now Vice President of the Colombian Social Security Institute. His research area is health sytems, with a particular focus on evaluation of policy, health reform (decentralisation, social security) and the comparative study of health systems. His recent publications include I. Jaramillo, G. Olano and F.J. Yepes (1998) *La ley 100. Cuatro años de implementación* (Bogotá: Editorial Guadalupe).

List of Tables

List of Illustrations

CHAPTER 1

Health Policy in Latin America: Themes, Trends and Challenges

Christopher Abel and Peter Lloyd-Sherlock

Through the 1980s and '90s, public policies in Latin America were the subject of increasing scrutiny and radical reforms. These processes of change were driven by economic crises in the 1980s and by a subsequent shift from state-led development to an almost unquestioning belief in neoliberalism. At the same time, international development banks took a growing interest in the 'social sectors' and had a significant influence on the direction of change.[1] In no area of policy were these processes more apparent than in health services. However, less has been written about health and healthcare in Latin America than for other aspects of social policy, and what has been written is mainly from a public health perspective which contributes little to broader social policy debates. To some extent, this reflects the disinclination of social scientists to study a field that is considered highly technical and the reluctance of clinical scientists to take a 'soft' approach to a subject which before the 1980s was largely viewed as the domain of public health specialists and physicians.

There are many reasons for taking a deeper academic interest in Latin American healthcare. The challenge of responding to demographic, epidemiological and technical changes must be put in a broader social, economic and political context. Furthermore, the health sector may itself have a major impact on social and economic development. As well as promoting welfare and human capital formation, healthcare is an industry and a major employer in its own right, connected with pharmaceutical companies, the insurance sector and equipment manufacturers. Health services account for between one third and one half of total social expenditure in most Latin American countries. However, the Pan American Healthcare Organisation (PAHO) has estimated that in the early 1990s around 130 million people in Latin America and the Caribbean had no access whatsoever to formal healthcare.[2] As such, the region remained a long way from achieving the 1978 Alma Ata Declaration of Health For All by the Year 2000.[3]

---

[1] In 1993 the flagship publication of the World Bank, *The World Development Report*, was entirely devoted to changing health systems (World Bank, 1993a). The following year, it published a major policy document on reforming pension programmes (World Bank, 1994).

[2] Mesa-Lago (1992).

[3] The Alma Ata Declaration, that all people in all countries have access to health (including psychological and social welfare) became the central strategy of the World Health Organisation and provided the impetus for primary healthcare programmes across the world (World Health Organisation, 1978).

Latin American healthcare systems and services display a number of distinctive features, which justify the regional focus taken in this book. Most systems suffer from a level of segmentation and a bias towards hospital care that is extreme even by developing country standards. Table 1.1 indicates that the richer Latin American countries devote relatively large amounts of funding to health, but that they do not compare well to other middle-income countries in terms of outputs and performance. The region has witnessed arguably the most radical set of neoliberal inspired health sector reforms in the world. These include the pioneering experiment of Chile in the early 1980s and more recent initiatives in Mexico and Argentina. Considerable diversity exists in the region, including Colombia's ambitious programme to develop a unified and universal health system and the singular success of socialist Cuba. Despite the persistence of the US trade embargo and the collapse of the USSR, the country is still among the top five per cent of developing countries in terms of social welfare indicators.

Table 1.1: Selected Health Statistics by World Region, c. 1990

	Total per capita health spend, 1990 (dollars)	Doctors per 1,000 population, 1988-92	Perinatal mortality rate per 1,000, 1990
Latin America	105	1.25	33
Former Socialist Economies	142	4.07	19
China	11	1.37	25
India	21	0.41	64
Other Asia	61	0.31	49
Established Market Economies	1,860	2.52	9

Source: World Bank (1993).

Latin America is also diverse in terms of its healthcare needs.[4] The larger cities of the Southern Cone contain aged populations and suffer high rates of chronic disease. Conversely, some rural districts of the poorer countries show no signs of entering any recognisable form of demographic or epidemiological transition and continue to experience very high levels of mortality (often from easily preventable conditions). The region has not been immune to the global re-emergence of infectious diseases such as tu-

---

[4] Pan American Health Organisation (1999).

berculosis (TB), nor to the appearance of new ones, such as HIV/AIDS. While there has been considerable success in controlling the cholera outbreaks of the early 1990s, progress with long-established diseases such as Chagas' or malaria has been negligible. More general improvements in population health ultimately depend on the capacity of macroeconomic policies to deliver an improved standard of living to the poorest and most vulnerable: as yet there are few signs that this is happening.

Health issues and healthcare systems are extremely diverse and highly complex, touching on a wide range of academic disciplines. It is vital to take a multi-sectoral approach, since factors such as income, education and housing may have as much impact on health outcomes as healthcare per se. Studying health policy may give us valuable insights into a range of other important debates, including good governance and the relationships between the public and private sectors. Clearly, it is beyond the scope of any single volume to deal with all of these questions in detail for a region as large and diverse as Latin America. This book (as did the conference out of which it arose) seeks to take a preliminary, exploratory approach and to highlight a number of key themes.

Before proceeding, a number of potential pitfalls in the use of health data should be identified. Table 1.1 provides a selection of health statistics for different world regions for around 1990. This sort of information can sometimes be of use for making very broad generalisations, but should be treated with extreme caution. First, and most obviously, such geographically aggregated data are bound to hide more than they reveal. The same is true of data given for individual countries, which often mask sharp internal variations. For example, the number of doctors per capita varied by almost ten-fold between different parts of Mexico in the late 1980s.[5] Second, great care must be taken when considering cause and effect. Standard health indicators, such as mortality rates, only give an extremely indirect view of the performance of health services, since they are determined by many additional factors, such as nutrition, housing and income. Likewise, measurements of healthcare infrastructure can sometimes be misleading. In many Former Socialist Economies there is a problem of over-supply of certain services, particularly trained medics, which waste resources and distort patterns of provision. Similar problems are evident in much of Latin America. A more fundamental difficulty is the reliability and completeness of the data for the region and technical and political flaws often compound problems of incomplete reporting.[6]

---

[5] McGreevey (1990).
[6] Perhaps surprisingly, Cuba is one of the few exceptions to this problem. Independent auditing checks have shown its vital statistic and health reporting systems to be among the most complete and accurate in the developing world.

Healthcare and the state

It is generally accepted that guaranteeing health for society as a whole should be a core responsibility of any state.[7] In Latin America there is huge diversity, both in terms of the overall nature of states and their relationships to social welfare.[8] These include:

1. The all-embracing welfare state under siege (notably Cuba).
2. The incomplete welfare state in retreat (observed in different contexts in Argentina and Nicaragua).
3. The 'restored' liberal democracy, for which economic growth and democratic consolidation are higher priorities than a social policy that is either coherent in conception or all-embracing in coverage (Chile and Brazil).
4. The disarticulated state in partial decomposition, as in Colombia, where healthcare resources have in places been distorted by conflict and violence.
5. The near-absent state that implicitly delegates social policy responsibilities to NGOs, such as Haiti.

Despite this diversity, over the past decade the region as a whole has experienced a trend towards the restoration of liberal democracy in some states and a drive to deepen democracy in others.[9] It is essential to understand how healthcare fits into this context of change. A key concern is how far Latin American states have broken habits of using health policy and delivery systems as instruments of political patronage, so that finances are regularised and so that vote-winning actions do not by necessity prevail over other considerations (for example, the construction of a new hospital is not by definition preferred to the maintenance of existing ones). In addition, it is useful to assess how open, honest and inclusive debates about healthcare reform have been. The book contains two examples (El Salvador and Argentina), which portray the reform process as relatively secretive and closed, despite a democratic rhetoric of accountability and transparency.

Discussion of public policy is often pervaded by an uncritical confidence among liberal professionals in the capacity of liberal democracy to achieve their goals. Some doubts should be expressed about over-optimistic equations between democratic government and better social services; of state reform and a reduction in clientelism; and of economic growth and positive health effects. We should not take it for granted that a consolidated liberal democracy intrinsically means better healthcare. It would be both misleading and retrograde to argue that more progress in healthcare has been usually achieved under dictatorships: in Haiti, the Dominican Republic and pre-revolutionary Nicaragua, abusive dictatorships were associated with

[7] Mackintosh (1992).
[8] Grindle (1996); Hartlyn and Morley (eds.) (1996); and Teitel (ed.) (1992).
[9] Ai Camp (ed.) (1995); Tulchin and Romero (eds.) (1995); and Dominguez and Lowenthal (eds.) (1996).

pitifully inadequate healthcare systems. Nevertheless, recent experience suggests that neither leftist nor centrist democratic parties have placed health issues boldly on their agendas and liberal democracies have often favoured the private sector at the expense of issues of public concern. Indeed, Venezuela, at times seen as the most durable example of effective liberal democracy in Latin America, has witnessed some of the most brutal and insensitive cuts in social policy spending in the continent.

In health, as in other spheres of public policy, attention must be paid to the capacity, competence and willingness of state agencies to implement policy and to meet their responsibilities. National health ministries may be constrained by constitutional or other statutory provisions that confine their role to setting norms, rather than enforcing them, and by competition between different levels of government and with other ministries also responsible for health issues. The continuing politicisation of posts and a high level of turnover of officials at the regional and local levels often frustrate even the routine performance of basic tasks, let alone innovative practice. Stressing 'accountability' may simply mean a higher level of turnover and greater emphasis on marketing policy, rather than a growth in competence.

Many Latin American republics have experienced a recent stress on local democratisation in which programmes of municipal reform and decentralisation have played an important part.[10] There would appear to be a regional (or even global) consensus that decentralisation can improve the quality, efficiency and responsiveness of health services, while deepening democratisation.[11] However, the evidence is variable and does not always support these claims.[12] Although the abstract logic of decentralising healthcare may appear to make sense, in the context of some Latin American states it can sometimes do more harm than good. In decentralised systems, policy formulated at the centre may not be applied in the locality or may be carried out in a diluted or distorted form for lack of human or fiscal resources.[13] Decentralisation may sometimes be little more than an all-purpose panacea for ministers and senior policy-makers, who are determined to be seen to be active but have few other ideas. Too easily, a policy of decentralisation can be an instrument for shunting off responsibilities for crucial issues like the supply of drinking water to local authorities that lack the funds and the competence to handle them. Health ministries in several countries have appointed advisers to help municipal government prepare plans and projects. But it is unlikely that there are enough advisers of sufficient quality to give more than routine assistance to the majority of municipalities. Where a few countries may have the resources to realise the objectives of municipal reform and decentralisation nationwide, the poorest clearly do not, and countries of intermediate ranking may have the re-

---

[10] Araujo Jr. (1997); Collins and Green (1994); and Nickson (1995).
[11] Cassels (1995).
[12] Rogers (1996), González-Block et al. (1989) and Cassels (1995) all question the supposed benefits of healthcare decentralisation in the region.
[13] Grindle and Thomas (eds.) (1991).

sources in some regions and cities, but not in others. In such countries, the overall impact of the policy will be to exacerbate disparities.

The roles of the public and private sectors

The potential of the public sector to develop an effective regulatory role, both for its own services and for the emergent private healthcare sector, is an issue of increasing concern. If the state has failed as a direct provider of health services, then it seems fair to question its capacity for regulating the activities of other actors. This is made more difficult by the high level inter-penetration of state and private sector interests in the region, both at the institutional level (for example, state subsidies for national drugs manufacturers) and at the individual one (government officials who also run private health clinics and consultancies). Timidity of the state in the face of the private sector is a recurring theme in this book. Health ministries and other state agencies often lack competent personnel to cope with an expanding range of problems of legitimate concern to the private healthcare sector, trade unions, peasant organisations and other representative bodies. Particular areas of interest include regulating private healthcare financiers and providers, as well as occupational and environmental health (ironically, outside the remit of the British National Health Service from its inception). This raises related questions of how far employers (including public sector agencies) can, especially in rural areas, resist or ignore state surveillance of health risks for lack of legislation or qualified personnel and even whether they are aware of state regulations.

At the centre of these debates is a concern with privatisation, or, perhaps, to put it better, a shift from public to private sector management. This process has affected all aspects of healthcare systems in Latin America, including financing and service provision. The Inter-American Development Bank estimates that by the mid-1990s private prepaid medical plans served almost 50 million people in the region, the great majority coming from high income groups.[14] Predictions that private insurance will continue to expand rapidly have aroused interest beyond the region. Latin America is now perceived as a major emerging market for US insurance firms and healthcare maintenance organisations.[15] Across the region, there is little debate about the virtue of embracing the US model of private healthcare, which has abjectly failed in its own country.

One aspect of privatisation that has received little attention in the general literature is the training of health professionals. Long admired by the World Bank and economic liberals as a paragon of low taxation, good debt management and freedom for entrepreneurial initiative, Colombia illustrates the risks associated with attaching a low priority to social policy over a long period in a context of turmoil and violence. Among other things, this has given rise to under-regulated private security and 'self-defence' groups,

---

[14] Inter-American Development Bank (1996).
[15] Stocker et al. (1999).

operating with few official constraints in the absence of an efficient police force. These problems are equally evident in the medical education sector, where controls over the development of new private faculties were increasingly relaxed during the late 1970s and early '80s. This trend was associated with the rise of a new business ethic and profitable opportunities offered by founding new private medical schools. It encouraged the proliferation of barely regulated schools, with inadequate laboratory facilities, poor-quality teaching and inferior access to hospitals for clinical training. Fears for a new generation of inferior medical graduates seem well grounded. Despite the promises of successive governments to improve the quality of health services, it is suspected that the calibre of medical graduates continues to slip. Professional and business interests have impeded even token attempts to restrain the proliferation of medical schools — three in the Caribbean city of Barranquilla alone, more in Bogotá than in Paris.

A further area of concern is the consequence of globalisation and transnationalisation for the health sector. A standard question of the 1960s that has long been submerged should be allowed to resurface in fresh form: How far is the health sector being reshaped around the requirements of the transnational pharmaceutical (and, perhaps, hospital equipment) industries?[16]

During the import-substitution industrialisation ascendancy of the 1950s and '60s,[17] numerous family-run pharmaceutical enterprises sprang up in the main manufacturing cities of Latin America. Nationalist strategies of developing generic drugs in large quantities and at low prices were mooted but seldom followed through. More recently, aggressive price liberalisation programmes have enlarged the range of pharmaceutical products, gone some way towards stabilising supplies and have simplified the role of the state. However, these policies have also had a range of negative effects. Overvalued exchange rates have reduced the cost of imported pharmaceuticals and, together with the liberalisation of import controls, the deregulation of product registration and the imposition of patent protection for chemicals developed overseas, they have undermined small domestic producers. In the poorest countries, pharmaceutical firms remain monopolistic, or at best oligopolistic, and any notion of competition is fictional. Yet, even where competition in the pharmaceutical sector is obviously absent, finance ministers, especially the more doctrinaire neoliberals, are likely to resist moves which hint at a revival of protectionism and regulation, let alone subsidies for the poor. In the medium term, particularly if national currencies are devalued, price liberalisations may well increase the cost of drugs, creating further budgetary problems for health ministries and reducing access for the poor. In addition, liberalisation can be blamed

---

[16] Gereffi (1983); Silverman (1976); and CEPAL (1987).

[17] Policies that place state-led industrialisation behind tariff boundaries at the centre of economic strategy. For an introduction, see Thorp in Abel and Lewis (1993).

for excessive promotion and advertising, along with over-consumption in a continent where entrenched traditions of self-prescription make for excessive usage: pharmaceuticals typically account for 25–30 per cent of healthcare budgets.[18] The scope for the introduction of new generic strategies, a potentially efficient option involving limited controls on specified drugs, is restricted in the current economic climate.

At the local level, long-standing reservations about the content and quality of information diffused to customers of pharmacies remain relevant. Until the middle of the century graduate pharmacists formulated and dispensed affordable pharmaceuticals in their shops. However, in recent decades pharmacies have increasingly shifted to the sale of pre-packaged drugs; and pharmacy graduates, once 'independent' professionals, have found that their only job outlets are as agents of the national and transnational pharmaceutical industries, so that little information from outside the industry is available to consumers.

Health, poverty and social exclusion

Increasing credence is being given to the view that investing in basic education and health services is the best way to reduce poverty in the developing world.[19] The development of appropriate health policies could go a long way to reducing the two-way relationship between poverty and ill health. However, entitlement and access to healthcare in most Latin American countries mirror the stratification and inequity of their societies as a whole, reinforcing rather than mitigating social divides. The policy responses are often obvious; it is more difficult to explain why they are so rarely put into practice. This can only be done by understanding the dynamics of poverty and exclusion across the region, how social problems are perceived and labelled and how perceptions change over time. Concepts such as social exclusion and vulnerability have come to the fore relatively recently, but should be viewed as only the latest in a succession of attempts to understand (and justify) the extent of social problems facing regions such as Latin America.[20]

In the 1910s and '20s liberal intelligentsias spoke of the 'social question' and some liberals moralised feverishly about how far visions of economic development were obstructed by a low-wage, low-productivity labour force of the 'undeserving poor', supposedly characterised by alcoholism, abject laziness, venereal diseases and poor nutritional habits. The Catholic Church and its corporatist allies appropriated the concept of 'social action' in the 1930s and '40s as their response to continuing poverty and misery. Piety, conformity and the strengthening of hierarchical bonds and the patriarchal family unit would lead, or so it was claimed, to moral redemption and would make possible the personal and social discipline necessary to generate an employable, adequately nourished workforce,

---

[18] Madrid et al. (1998).
[19] Morley (1995).
[20] De Kadt (1994).

while engendering a habit of small savings.[21] The concept of 'social justice' gained some momentum from the 1940s. In a period of accelerating urbanisation it had a manifest appeal to elements of the lower middle class and organised labour, which supported governments in exchange for social 'interventions' that provided some guarantee against illness and unemployment and that mitigated hardships in the troughs of economic cycles. However, as evidence mounted across Latin America that large swathes of the population, especially in the countryside, had slender or no access to even low-quality social services, despite decades of promises of 'social action' and 'social justice', 'social revolution' emerged as a viable and enduring concept. It was proclaimed with greatest commitment in revolutionary Cuba, but also enjoyed considerable purchase elsewhere. Temporarily in abeyance in government circles since the Nicaraguan counter-revolution, the theme of 'social revolution' is still to be heard among radical movements of the rural poor in Mexico and Brazil.

Concepts such as social exclusion and vulnerability raise various problems of definition. We need to distinguish those groups excluded from all social services from those excluded from one but not estranged from another (health but not education) from those excluded from good-quality services. Secondly, we need to distinguish families and households where some members are excluded from the benefits of official provision from those where all are. Thirdly, we need to distinguish the long-term excluded from the once included and newly excluded and dispossessed: uprooted internal migrants in Colombia; refugees from Nicaragua elsewhere in Central America; and the victims of disasters, like Hurricane Mitch in Honduras and Nicaragua. We need, finally, to identify the self-excluded, who opt in preference for the services of the traditional healer or midwife.

Here a mental picture of the urban household excluded from all aspects of social provision impinging on health may be of assistance. Such a household may be the victim of a cumulative series of social insults: the closure of a popular hospital, the delegation of its functions to ineffective health posts and exclusion from the price benefits of streamlined food supplies through modern supermarket chains, exclusion from a clean drinking water-supply caused by the unwillingness of a privatised supplier to operate in loss-making slums. If social exclusion is, in some instances, becoming a more acute problem, then some broader questions of ideology and policy arise. How far does a democratic strengthening imply notions of citizenship that go beyond civil liberties to embrace social rights? Have 'new social movements' succeeded in incorporating once excluded kin and neighbourhood networks, or have their leaders been co-opted and much of their followings re-excluded?

---

[21] Ivereigh (1995).

Health and violence

In recent decades, Latin America has experienced little of the international warfare that has plagued other developing regions, but it has been subjected to high levels of political and social violence and also of criminality. Estimates for Brazil have indicated that three people are murdered every hour, with 67.3 officially reported murders per 100,000 inhabitants in Rio de Janeiro during 1992.[22] Domestic violence is increasingly being recognised as a key health policy issue in the region. A recent survey of women in Managua (Nicaragua) found that over half had experienced some form of abuse, as defined by PAHO. These women had suffered significant losses of earnings and made twice as much use of healthcare services as did other women.[23]

In various countries high indices of crime, domestic violence and road accidents have been complemented by armed violence by the agents and allies of governments, by guerrillas and paramilitaries and by networks of narcotics and armaments dealers. Psychological violence connected with torture, disappearances and forced migration has also occurred. Orphans and traumatised, abandoned and immunologically weak children, some of them street children persecuted by vigilantes in cities like Rio de Janeiro, São Paulo and Cali, have been victims too. With political violence the physical infrastructure of healthcare has been dislocated and destroyed; the vigilance and control of transmissible diseases have been significantly disrupted; the movement of equipment in vaccination campaigns has been delayed (or the campaigns postponed) and personnel displaced.[24]

Violence can lead to a shrinking of coverage and an 'atomisation' of health programmes; it can provide a pretext for reducing costs by excluding populations in areas of conflict. In several countries hospital resources have been diverted from routine operations to the casualties of violence. In some cases, resources allocated to primary care have been transferred to tertiary care and rehabilitation. Similarly, violence frequently signifies the disruption of the food supply and its appropriation by soldiers or guerrillas, the eviction or flight of rural populations, bad harvests and breakdowns in systems of distribution. These may have inflationary and nutritional consequences for the poor and, in particular, for the dispossessed and displaced, who are also exposed to infectious diseases.

In some areas of violence, doctors and nurses have themselves been political actors. Denounced by the Contras in Nicaragua as disguised military advisers, Cuban aid workers were sometimes singled out as targets.[25] More recently, in some Andean countries doctors and nurses have strongly voiced their disillusionment about the quality of official healthcare in the hospitals and health posts of violent frontier zones. Some, rejecting the official ap-

---

[22] Flynn (1993).
[23] Morrison and Orlando (1997).
[24] Ugalde and Zwi (eds.)(1994).
[25] Garfield (1989).

propriation of medical language (for example, the 'virus of communism'), continue to join guerrilla movements. The memory of the Argentine doctor who took part in the Cuban revolutionary struggle, Ernesto 'Che' Guevara, continues to have some appeal and resonance.

Health professionals

An issue that has attracted scant attention in recent decades is the appropriateness of western medical education to Latin American conditions. As early as the late 1940s and '50s, the displacement of the French ascendancy in medical education by that of the United States raised anxieties about the stress on an expensive, curative, high-technology medicine and the downgrading in some countries of preventive concerns and some areas of 'tropical medicine'. The curricula content and priorities of many medical faculties are much better geared to prosperous surgeries and middle-class patients than to underfunded health posts and the poor. When a surplus of doctors and nurses exists to serve the requirements of the upper and middle classes, inappropriate training may foster professional emigration to North America and Western Europe. Across Latin America, medical faculties have produced too many specialists pursuing prestigious employment and too few general practitioners. In some districts doctors should be trained to cope with conditions where villagers combine elements of diverse therapeutic traditions pragmatically.[26] Also, there are few signs that medical anthropology has been integrated effectively into medicine curricula, as envisaged 20 years ago.

In most Organisation for Economic Cooperation and Development (OECD) countries there are three or four trained nurses for every physician. In Mexico, their numbers are roughly equal, while in Argentina and Colombia there are several doctors for every nurse. An acute shortage of trained nurses compounds the problems caused by a lack of generalist physicians. The preponderance of doctors wastes resources through a top-heavy wage structure and reinforces the bias towards specialist hospital-based care. It is difficult to identify a clear explanation for this imbalance in human resources. Contributing factors include the failure of states to regulate private medical schools and a deep-seated belief that medical treatment from a nurse is inherently inferior. Indeed, nursing remains a low status activity across the region, particularly in the public sector, where salaries and working conditions are often appalling.[27]

A related issue is the geographical distribution of health professionals. The case for all graduates undertaking a year of rural service is, of course, a strong one. But it presumes a quality of public administration, which is only too often absent. During the 1930s, Mexico pioneered the concept of the 'rural year' in Latin America, by which every newly graduated physician was required to spend one year ministering to the needs of villagers

---

[26] Brodwin (1996).
[27] Stillwaggon (1998).

before being formally qualified.[28] Emulated in rural Colombia in the 1950s, and later extended to slum areas in Bogotá, Cali and elsewhere, the year of social service was so poorly administered by the late 1980s that the Medical Faculty of the National University was sometimes compelled to improvise positions for its outgoing students as keepers of instruments, so that they might comply with the legal requirement to undertake a social service before entering full-time professional practice. This occurred because the Public Health Ministry did not have the administrative competence to create positions for young men and women in areas — rural or urban — of greatest medical need. Likewise in rural Ecuador, despite the presence of a similar programme, only 30 per cent of births were attended by a health professional by the mid-1990s.[29]

Healthcare reforms

Readers should beware of the overuse of the term 'reform'. Most governments have a tendency to market all changes as 'reforms' and many ministers wish to be seen to be undertaking new and far-reaching reform projects, rather than consolidating existing schemes. Healthcare systems in all Latin American countries have, throughout their existence, been subject to continuous attempts at reform, most of which were never implemented. However, the 1990s have seen an intensification of the reform process across the region. Particular emphasis has been given to a shift in the private-public sector mix in finance, the development of new management strategies and policies of decentralisation. At the same time, the concepts of equity and efficiency have come to the fore.

The increased attention paid to equity reflects a concern that public spending in general and health spending in particular are often markedly regressive.[30] However, the prominence given to equity may be, in part, because it is a concept around which social democrats, liberals and conservatives can build a consensus. The notion of a 'progress towards equity' does not offend or challenge propertied interests as a stress on equality does; and indeed, a 'progress towards equity' may be fast or slow to the point of being barely perceptible. Moreover, equity is extremely hard to define or measure and can be understood from a range of philosophical viewpoints.[31]

The stress on equity may mean that past commitments to protect the weak citizen from market dependency and past objectives of universal welfare have been compromised. If this has occurred, should it be viewed as a more realistic and pragmatic approach to health policy or a retrenchment of welfare? To what extent has it been associated with the retreat from a notion of healthcare as an entitlement of citizenship

---

[28] Nigenda (1997).

[29] Inter-American Development Bank (1996).

[30] Lloyd-Sherlock (2000).

[31] Mooney (1987) provides an excellent review of different philosophical approaches to social equity, including entitlement, utilitarian and egalitarian.

rather than as a privilege or commodity? In areas of acute poverty, where the market economy is especially weak, a view of healthcare as a commodity is especially questionable.

When seeking ways to promote equity in Latin America, a key consideration has to be the segmentation of healthcare systems. In much of the region social security programmes account for almost as much health expenditure as the public sector, but often only provide for a relatively privileged minority of the population.[32] Social security programmes usually capture a number of substantial indirect subsidies from the state sector, such as the training of doctors and the dumping of chronic or expensive conditions on public hospitals. In some countries the situation has been extended by the emergence of a significant private insurance sector, which sometimes works alongside social security programmes and sometimes competes against them.[33]

In the new wave of healthcare reforms, equity concerns have gone hand in hand with debates over the efficiency of healthcare systems. During the 1980s it became apparent that health services had been extended with insufficient regard to issues of cost or effectiveness.[34] In 1985 the World Health Organisation (WHO) Regional Committee for the Americas estimated that around 30 per cent of health spending in Latin America was wasted.[35] A separate study calculated that between ten and 30 per cent of hospital treatments performed were of no clinical value.[36] The most widely cited example of this is the overuse of caesarian sections, with rates of 50 per cent or higher in several countries, notably Brazil.

This range of issues explains, at least in part, why health policy has increasingly become the domain of economists, finance ministries and new 'entrepeneurial' managers (as evidenced by the recent appearance of MSc courses in health administration in several Latin American countries). In their wake have come cost-benefit analyses and other forms of economic evaluation, which some consider to be a magic bullet for all the ills of social and economic policies.[37] These saw their clearest expression with the 1993 World Development Report, still the prime reference work for health economists working in developing countries. One particular concern has been to develop more 'sustainable' sources of revenue, which generally involve the promotion of private insurance and the implementation of user fees. Both of these policies are empirically unproven in the Latin American context and the few studies published to date disagree about their appropriateness.[38] Moreover, there

---

[32] Lloyd-Sherlock (2000).

[33] Barrientos and Lloyd-Sherlock (forthcoming, 2000).

[34] World Bank (1989).

[35] World Health Organisation (1985).

[36] Banta (1988).

[37] In fact, the use of cost-benefit analysis in planning health services at the national level goes back at least as far as the 1960s, when the PAHO/Centre for Development Studies (CENDES) programme in Venezuela attempted to operationalise a model which aimed to minimise deaths (taken as a crude indicator of health benefit) from a fixed health budget (Ahumada, 1965).

[38] Gertler et al. (1989); Gilson, Russel and Buse (1995); and La Forgia (1989).

are few signs that the most fundamental causes of inefficiency of healthcare services have been addressed by these developments. Healthcare systems across the region continue to suffer from an extreme curative and urban bias, inappropriate staffing structures and poorly coordinated, fragmented administrations. Also, the new economic imperative does little to resolve what is doubtless the largest source of health services inefficiency: ineffectual regulation and widespread corruption. It is unlikely that many Latin American states will be able to benefit from a drive towards efficiency without a thorough administrative reform that introduces and generalises Weberian concepts of administrative neutrality and that eliminates both clientelism and high levels of turnover of public officials. Nor is it likely that relatively high levels of health spending will lead to improved health indicators until significant reductions in income inequality are also obtained.

The rise of the health economist is paralleled by the changing fortunes of the different international organisations interested in health policy. The influence and impact of the World Health Organisation (WHO) and its Latin American sub-division the Pan-American Health Organisation (PAHO), along with the United Nations Educational, Scientific and Cultural Organisation (UNESCO) and the International Labour Organisation (ILO), has diminished in relative terms during the 1980s and '90s. Over the same time, the voices of the World Bank and the Inter-American Development Bank (IADB) have grown. The former organisations traditionally championed the 'Health for All' and primary healthcare movements of the 1970s. The latter have promoted the new wave of neoliberal inspired health sector reforms across the region. In some countries, these organisational divisions and cultures are mirrored in government, with health ministries retaining close links with the WHO, finance ministries with the banks and social security agencies with the ILO. The diminishing relative influence of PAHO (and its growing ties with the World Bank) may mean that non-governmental organisations (NGOs), with their broadening of activities to embrace themes of absolute poverty, have become the principal opposition to the neoliberal orthodoxy in social policy. Several contributors to this volume refer to resistance to recent reforms. Some reasons for resistance to reforms are evident: that assumptions widely prevalent among officials are not widely shared by junior professionals or public opinion (for example, an often doctrinaire assumption that the private sector is by definition more efficient than the public one; the belief that levels of taxation are too high even for the highest-income groups, even given problems of evasion; an assumption that taxation has only a small redistributive function; and an orthodoxy that 'downsizing' of public provision is desirable). Only too readily 'reformers' explain the failure to convert large numbers of patients and other users of health services to reform in terms of a failure to explain policies to public opinion or to carry out political analysis prior to reform.[39] Only too frequently 'reformers' are blind to the fact that vulnerable sections of the population have little confidence in reforms which are shaped from outside, and whose main impetus frequently comes from the fiscal imperatives of federal government rather than a desire to improve and extend services.

Despite the shift in reform priorities, upgrading primary healthcare services is still on the agenda for some Latin American countries. Indeed, the adjustment policies of the 1980s and early '90s may have forced some governments into overdue reappraisals of priorities and restored, if only rhetorically, an emphasis on primary health. However, this may have been driven by fiscal imperatives, and especially a stress on cost reductions, as much as by broader considerations of the eradication of poverty and inequality.[40]

Calls for less emphasis on the hospital sector and the devolution of resources to primary health posts are hardly new. As early as the 1930s, public health reformers called for a reallocation of resources to local health units, particularly to deal with the health of mothers and infants, whom it was felt imprudent to expose to the then considerable risks of contracting diseases in charity and public hospitals. Yet hospitals remain resilient institutions, with considerable bargaining strength in struggles over budgets. Officials demanding a shift from funding of hospitals to primary health posts sometimes forget that local hospitals are symbols of successful past struggles, involving trade unions, junior professionals and government agencies, and are usually regarded with affection even where the quality of their services is not uniformly good.

A key objective of primary healthcare has been to 'enlist the poor' in community decisions — there has been less emphasis on 'enlisting the rich' and their role as responsible citizens. However, it is of little surprise that populations exposed on a daily basis to the rhetoric of accountability and consultation have more confidence in sceptical views expressed by nurses and physicians, whom they meet on a regular basis, than in politicians and bureaucrats. Many health professionals see the consequences of neoliberal policies on a daily basis, and recall the slowness with which policies designed to mitigate the most severe effects have been drawn up and implemented.

The chapters in this volume

The book begins with a general proposal for a new approach to healthcare systems, which, it is claimed, could be applied in most Latin American countries. Londoño and Frenk's model of 'structured pluralism' sets out a blueprint for a new arrangement in which the private and public sectors collaborate in the pursuit of equity, market contestability and allocational efficiency. Londoño and Frenk are anxious to avoid what they perceive as

---

[39] The form of political analysis currently in vogue is known as 'stakeholder analysis'. Glassman et al. (1999) apply this approach to health reform proposals in the Dominican Republic.
[40] Abel and Lewis (eds.) (1993); Bulmer-Thomas (ed.) (1996); and Berry (ed.) (1998).

the extremes of authoritarian controls and a monopolistic denial of choice to patients in the public sector, and the atomisation and lack of structures found in the private one. They propose a specifically Latin American model, which is distinct from European public contracts, Canadian provider autonomy and US managed competition.

In the structured pluralism model the role of the health ministry would primarily be one of 'modulation', in which it sets transparent and fair rules throughout both the private and public sectors. Health financing would become the essential function of social security institutes and New Organisations for Health Services would be responsible for the management of care and organisation of networks of providers. The authors identify the risk that an incomplete application of this model would add a new segment to an already over-segmented healthcare system, instead of achieving a comprehensive approach to 'structured pluralism'. But they are open to other questions. Can a model designed for Latin America as a whole embrace the diversity of healthcare traditions and socioeconomic conditions in the region? Furthermore, the model has no overtly political dimension and so it does not set out to give practical proposals for the consultation of actors whose resistance might impede its implementation. Thus, the model has considerable merits, particularly as a stimulus for debate, but it should not be taken as a definite blueprint for policy.

Núria Homedes and her colleagues suggest that too many plans and projects are drawn up and too few fully implemented. They argue that reform should be anchored in national 'culture'. They also raise questions about how far reform efforts are moving satisfactorily in practice, whether they are more evident on paper and whether orthodoxies of 'downsizing' are compatible with a language of participation and accountability. Homedes and her colleagues mention the preference of the World Bank for working with agencies with which its staff are already familiar and, in particular, its preference for working with autonomous government agencies on the grounds that they are more efficacious and responsive than ministries. Further study could usefully explore how far this emphasis has negative consequences that are already manifest: encouraging a wasteful duplication of effort and a destructive competition for prestige and resources between agencies with overlapping functions.

Homedes et al. go on to look at these issues with reference to a recent healthcare reform initiative in El Salvador. This process was led by the World Bank, along with a special Health Reform Group set up as a separate entity from the Ministry of Health. The authors characterise the reform process as highly secretive — indeed they were themselves unable to obtain basic items of information. The proposals followed a standard neoliberal approach: a combination of privatisation, decentralisation and some selective primary healthcare initiatives. Homedes et al. point out contradictions in the reform process, including its purported goal of promoting participation in health policy, while suppressing debate about the reform itself. However, before implementation could begin, disagreements between the national government and the World Bank led to the collapse of the reform process.

The difficulties of implementing 'rational' healthcare reforms at the micro level are clearly depicted in Sarah Atkinson's chapter on decentralisation in the north-east of Brazil. Looking at three different districts within the state of Ceará, she finds considerable variation in patterns of interpretation and implementation of the national reform programme. These largely reflect the complex micro-political dynamics operating in each district, including the degree to which clientelism or *coronelismo* influences local health policy and the different perspectives and attitudes of health professionals. Atkinson draws attention to the limitations of short and superficial fact-finding visits by foreigners, observing that Brazilians are very adept at presenting policy and practice in a way which satisfies international norms and models, even if the reality is often very far from this. The same could be said about most other Latin American countries. This tendency often involves an element of collusion between international agencies, which are not prepared to probe or see what they are not meant to see (or what does not fit within their particular agendas). The development of appropriate health policies needs researchers who are familiar with the region and who do not gloss over the 'messiness' of local contexts.

Despite these barriers, sweeping health reforms are sometimes implemented largely as planned. This would appear to have been the case in Chile during the Pinochet dictatorship. The absence of any form of democratic process helped to speed up the reform process and prevented any significant modification of the original project as it was put into practice. However, it also precluded debate or participation in the reform process and gave rise to policies which some argue have been detrimental to the majority of the population. Too often, accounts of healthcare reforms in Chile fall into the trap of taking sides in the ideological debates about neo-liberalism. Left-wing critics are inclined to label every aspect of the changes as iniquitous.[41] Conversely, the development banks and free-marketeers portray the Institutos de Salud Previsional (ISAPREs) as a partly flawed but redeemable policy initiative, much of which could serve as a model for Latin America and beyond.[42] The chapter by Barrientos avoids either of these approaches and gives a cautious, objective appraisal of the initial reforms and the modifications made to them under subsequent democratic administrations. He observes that the first set of changes sought to promote the participation of private health insurance funds and to decentralise public services through the 'municipalisation' of primary healthcare. In many respects, the reforms succeeded in these objectives, although Barrientos argues that their principal impact was to increase segmentation, with private insurers attracting high income groups and state programmes increasingly

---

[41] Trumper and Phillips (1997).
[42] World Bank (1993a).

becoming an insurer (if not a provider) of last resort. During the 1990s
there were attempts to shore up the public healthcare sector, with particular
efforts to ensure a satisfactory level of service to poorer groups. However,
the basic structures established in the 1980s still remain and Barrientos asks
how the continuing division between private and state provision can be justified either in terms of efficiency or equity.

Cuba is, of course, a special, and, in public health, a most interesting
case. Garfield and Holtz outline the problems that a health system erected
in the 1960s and '70s, built upon socialist assumptions of universality of access from cradle to grave, has confronted in the face of a sustained US embargo, the collapse of the Soviet Union and domestic economic crisis.
Falling protein and caloric intakes have contributed to the under-nutrition
associated with outbreaks of optic neurotherapy, which placed new strains
on a public health budget already over-stretched by, for example, the
problem of rising costs of improved drugs as the *peso* lost value. Meanwhile, deteriorating housing and a decline in sanitary conditions and access
to a clean water supply contributed to a reappearance of tuberculosis.

From the 1960s free healthcare, like free education, was a means by
which the revolutionary regime led by President Fidel Castro won popular legitimacy. And physicians and nurses played an important part in
sustaining popular opposition to the United States by stressing that the
embargo embraced even pharmaceuticals, medicaments and hospital
equipment required urgently by children. In the 1970s a surplus of
nurses and doctors that was exported as part of aid programmes to Nicaragua, Angola and elsewhere was invaluable to the regime for propaganda
purposes in Latin America and Africa. And a domestic biotechnology programme gained some momentum in the 1980s. Yet by the mid-1990s
Cuba had ceased to be a net exporter of healthcare. Hampered by breakdowns in electric energy and shortages of spare parts for hospital equipment, the health system lurched from crisis to crisis. Yet it survived.

Thus, the problems that confronted Cuba were not those of the
mainland liberal regimes. A high level of equity had been achieved; and
efficiency was evident in successes in the 1990s in targeting that secured
a continuing decline in death rates of mothers and children. However,
as the private sector grew in other areas of activity in Cuba, so too did
inequalities of income, so that doctors and nurses came to figure among
low-income groups, by comparison, for example, with private farmers.
And professional morale sagged further.

Cuba's success in extending health provision to the poor is a stark contrast
to the situation in most Latin America countries. Gómez-Dantés provides a
frank critique of a recent attempt to extend healthcare coverage to the poor
in Mexico. The Programme for the Extension of Coverage (PEC) was instituted in 1996 and aims to ensure that ten million Mexicans previously without any access to formal care receive a minimum package of basic
interventions. Gómez-Dantés puts PEC in the broader context of Mexican

health reforms, noting that any benefits in terms of equity will be more than outweighed by a major increase of government financing for the privileged social security sector. He argues that the resources being devoted to PEC and the way in which it has been developed mean that it will only have a minimal impact on the health of the poor. The chapter makes the pertinent observation that reform which benefits the poor is only politically acceptable under a number of circumstances: when it does not divert resources from other groups with more capacity to mobilise politically; when it does not offend entrenched professional interests; and when it is financed by an external loan (in this case, World Bank money) rather than tax increases. Gomez-Dantés also notes that evaluations of the PEC have been minimal and that they have not been made publicly available: this would seem to contradict the World Bank's stated policy goal of promoting accountable government.

Lloyd-Sherlock's chapter investigates the history of failure to bring about systematic reform of healthcare in Argentina. By the first decades of the twentieth century there already existed haphazard, unregulated networks of mutual associations and 'health firms'. The degree of fragmentation of services that Lloyd-Sherlock depicts is perhaps not as surprising as he presents it. Absence of coordination was just as apparent in British, French and US provision before the First World War. However, in Argentina the main elements of this organisational structure were allowed to continue until the early 1990s, with trade unions having appropriated the management of most health funds. The weaknesses of this system in terms of cost, quality, coverage, equity and the unsystematic cross-subsidisation of the private and public sectors were evident by the 1970s and '80s; and health was often seen as an element of negotiation between trade unions and the government rather than as a goal in itself.

In the 1990s the government of Carlos Menem obtained lavish external funding for a new reform programme. Indeed, officials from poorer countries might, with reason, query why the international agencies, usually complaining of their own lack of resources, have been so generous in assisting a relatively rich society. Lloyd-Sherlock outlines Argentine proposals for a transition from union funds to a new model of flexible, consumer-led private provision, together with decentralisation of the public sector and an emphasis on training general practitioners. He expresses doubts about the implementation of a new regulatory framework and the effectiveness of a safety net for market failures in an environment where a culture of de-regulation pervades the highest echelons of the federal bureaucracy.

Colombia's health reforms provide in some respects a case opposite to that of Argentina. According to Yepes, this reform process has responded to several factors: an awareness of deficiencies of coverage and quality of the healthcare; a stress on political decentralisation and municipal reform; and the Constitution of 1991 (the first in Colombia since 1886), which proposes the principle that social security should be a right of all citizens. These reforms have two main thrusts. First, they seek to establish a unified and universal national health insurance scheme, which will include low-income groups who are unable to pay contributions. Second, they delegate responsibilities and resources to municipal governments. Many elements of the new system correspond closely to Frenk and Londoño's model of structured pluralism.

The reforms are ambitious and imaginative and, on paper at least, could do much to improve the lot of poor and vulnerable social sectors. Their immediate impact has apparently been positive, but it remains to be seen how successful they will be in the long run. For example, the reforms seek to assemble information on the financial capacity to pay of the entire population, but do the resources exist to update the database? Moreover, what is the quality of expertise in the Health Ministry, and are there sufficient consultants to supply more than routine assistance to the 1,080 municipalities that are entitled to draw up local health plans? Might decentralisation funding be appropriated by established political bosses, or serve as bases of patronage for new ones? Does not the problem of political and social dislocation — political violence in all departments and large numbers of internal refugees — pose significant obstacles to the normal functioning of the health sector, let alone the implementation of bold reform strategies? Yepes seeks to answer many of these questions, but they can only be fully resolved by complementary studies at the local level in both cities and the countryside. One fear is that the healthcare reform might suffer a similar fate to the Colombian Campaign against Absolute Poverty (1986–90). This was coherent, well conceived, carefully formulated and intelligently advocated, but ultimately collapsed due to a lack of sustained support from the president and the ruling party and its failure to achieve credibility among the poorest groups for whom it was intended.[43] In short, is the reform heroic, but divorced from reality, or does it represent a dramatic break with the past, and could it become an inspirational model for other countries in the region?

---

[43] Puyana (1993).

CHAPTER 2

Structured Pluralism:
Towards an Innovative Model for
Health System Reform in Latin America

Juan Luis Londoño
Julio Frenk

Introduction

Health systems are at a crossroads. Throughout the world there is a search for better ways to regulate, finance and deliver health services. There is a sense of impending innovation as countries at all levels of economic development, and with all types of political systems, engage in reform processes. Although the final outcome is still uncertain, it is possible that this search will lead to new conceptual and practical models for health systems.

This chapter seeks to develop options for restructuring health systems. In particular, it attempts to examine the shortcomings of present models and to advance an alternative. Our approach is both systematic — in that it analyses every element within a coherent framework — and systemic — in that it looks at the entire health system, with emphasis on the *relationships* among its major components. In today's complex environment, most problems tend to be interrelated. As a consequence, solutions cannot be focused only on one aspect of the health system while ignoring the rest. For example, if reforms are limited to decentralising services without changing the financing mechanisms, the incentives or the criteria for setting priorities, one is likely simply to multiply the problems of the previously centralised system. Such problems demand comprehensive approaches that deal with the health system as a whole. Because present failures are systemic, the reform response must also be systemic.

While the issues raised here are of interest to both wealthy and poor countries, we will mostly refer to Latin America. We are aware that generalisations are hampered by the enormous heterogeneity among and within the countries of the region. In fact, this analysis will emphasise the need to develop policies that take into account the diverse conditions coexisting in the region. To a large extent, social and economic inequality explain the mixed picture of health challenges in Latin America, where the problems of both the very rich and the very poor countries of the world are juxtaposed. This inequality is reflected in and reproduced by the heterogeneity of healthcare institutions, which have responded to the needs of the different social groups in a fragmented way.

The chapter will begin with a brief analysis of the main challenges facing the population and the healthcare institutions in Latin America. We will then propose a conceptualisation of the health system based on a series of key relationships and functions. This framework will serve to identify and compare the main existing models for organising the health system and the options for reforming them. Having analysed the limitations of extreme alternatives, we will develop a model of structured pluralism as a balanced approach to health system reform. We will also examine what appears to be a convergence towards this model. In order to move towards questions of implementation, the chapter will then discuss the main policy instruments that are available to carry forth the reform process. Finally, we will look at the strategies to increase the political feasibility of reforms.

The dual character of challenges

Many Latin American countries today face multiple opportunities stemming from advances in economic reform and democratisation. At the same time, however, these societies have to contend with complex challenges, which to a large extent derive from the rapid transformations of the post-war era. During the last half century, many Latin American countries have experienced changes that currently developed countries underwent over longer periods of time. This rapid modernisation has occurred at very different paces among the various segments of society, thereby increasing inequality among them.

Figure 2.1: Challenges to Health Systems in Latin America

COMPONENT	TYPE OF CHALLENGE	
	Accumulated	**Emerging**
Populations	- **Epidemiological backing** * Common infections * Malnutrition * Reproductive health problems - **Health gap** - **Inequity**	- **New Pressures** * Non-communicable diseases * Injuries * Emerging infections - **Changes in demand patterns** - **Political pressures**
Institutions	- **Insufficient coverage** - **Poor technical quality** - **Allocational inefficiency** - **Inadequate patient referral** - **Deficient management of institutions**	- **Cost escalation** - **Inadequate incentives** - **Financial insecurity** - **Patient dissatisfaction** - **Technological expansion** - **Deficient management of the system**

The combination of rapid and unequal change in many Latin American countries has brought them face to face with a series of new problems — characteristic of the more developed societies — without having totally solved the old problems — typical of poorer societies. Hence, past and future clash in a complex present. This is reflected in the juxtposition of a backlog of accumulated problems and a series of emerging challenges. Due to inequality, each set of challenges affects the various social groups and geographic areas differently.

In the health field, this duality is pervasive. As will be explained in the following section, every analysis of the health situation must look at two key elements: populations and institutions. For each of them, Figure 2.1 lists the two types of challenges. The empirical documentation of each challenge is beyond the scope of this chapter. Nevertheless, it is worth pointing out some of their key aspects.

Population-side challenges

Challenges affecting the population reflect the demographic and epidemiologic dynamics of the region. Other studies have examined these patterns of transition[1] and new projections of the burden of disease are available.[2] From the empirical evidence, it is clear that Latin America still suffers from an important epidemiological backlog represented by common infectious diseases, malnutrition and reproductive health problems.

Table 2.1: The Health Gap in Latin America and the Caribbean, c. 1995

Indicator	Observed Level	Expected Level	Gap
Health services coverage (% of the population)	78	89	14
Under-five mortality (per 1,000 births)	47	39	17%
Life-expectancy at birth (years)	69.5	72	4%
Burden of disease and injury (lost disability-adjusted life years per 1,000 persons)	231.6	200.1	14%

Source: Inter-American Development Bank (1996), pp. 242–3

The persistence of these problems reflects a gap between what would be potentially *achievable* under optimal performance and what is actually *achieved* by current health systems. One way of ascertaining this gap is to estimate the health situation that could be expected in a region given its level of development and compare such expectation with the observed conditions. A recent report by the Inter-American Development Bank offers empirical evidence about the gaps in different areas of social policy, including health.[3] Table 2.1 summarises that evidence. The observed values of

---

[1] Frenk, Bodadilla and Lozano (1996).
[2] Murray and Lozano (1996).
[3] Inter-American Development Bank (1996).

four indicators in Latin America and the Caribbean are compared to the levels that would be expected as a function of income per capita across the world. As can be seen, the observed health situation in Latin America and the Caribbean falls below expectation. The optimistic tone of many official reports is sobered by the realisation of this persistent gap, which becomes even more pronounced when one considers the inequities that characterise almost every Latin American country.[4]

Without having solved the accumulated challenges, the population of Latin America is already facing a set of emerging pressures (Figure 2.1). The demographic 'ageing' produced by the rapid decline in fertility, the accelerated process of urbanisation, the degradation of the environment and the adoption of unhealthy lifestyles are all responsible for a growing burden from non-communicable diseases and from injury. In addition, health systems have to meet the challenges of new infections, such as AIDS, or of re-emerging diseases that had been largely controlled in the past, such as malaria, dengue fever, cholera and tuberculosis.

To complicate the picture further, health systems are increasingly called upon to deal with the consequences of several forms of social disintegration, including war, displacement of populations and the expanding trade and consumption of illicit drugs.[5] Perhaps as a reflection of these processes, Latin America is experiencing a rapid growth in neuropsychiatric disorders, which have reached a prevalence of 10.18 per 100,000 persons, 56 per cent higher than the world average of 6.53 per 100,000. The prominence of neuropsychiatric disorders is a distinctive feature of the epidemiological transition in the region. This problem is compounded by a disproportionally high toll of violence. Latin America is the region with the highest burden of homicides, with a rate of 7.7 per 1,000 persons, which is more than twice the world average of 3.5 per 1,000. Recent estimates indicate that there are more than 100,000 homicides per year in Latin America, compared to 30,000 in all the industrialised countries.[6]

The epidemiological dynamics of the region are having complex effects on the overall demand for health services. The fertility decline will be reflected in a relative reduction of the demand for maternal and child health services, although this effect will take some years to develop fully in light of the 'demographic momentum', whereby the decline in the absolute *number* of births lags with respect to the reduction in the fertility *rate*, since there is a larger number of women of child-bearing age who were born under previous conditions of higher fertility.[7] Likewise, the increase in demand due to the ageing of the population takes time to express itself fully. What seems certain is that in the next decade the region will witness a generalised increase in the demand for health serv-

---

[4] Frenk, Bodadilla and Lozano (1996).
[5] Desjarlais et al. (1995).
[6] Londoño and Moser (1996).
[7] Bobadilla et al. (1993).

ices, although this process will be marked by the profound heterogeneity that exists among and within countries.

Another emerging pressure on the population side is the extension of democracy throughout the continent, which is likely to lead to growing political pressures for better and more diversified services,[8] as societies increasingly include healthcare among their basic citizenship rights.[9]

Institutional challenges

As can be seen, Latin America is experiencing an alignment of forces all of which point in the direction of growing pressures on health systems. Yet, as Figure 2.1 shows, the institutions that make up such systems are themselves subject to the duality of accumulated and emerging challenges. Thus, most countries in the region have not fully addressed age-old problems characteristic of less developed systems, such as insufficient coverage, poor technical quality, allocational inefficiency, inadequate processes for patient referral and deficient management of specific organisations.

At the same time, Latin America is already facing many of the issues that confound the more developed systems, such as cost escalation, incentives that run counter to the objectives of the system, financial insecurity, patient dissatisfaction, technological expansion and the many problems of managing the system as a whole over and above its specific organisations, including the challenges posed by growing pluralism.

The existing institutional fragmentation, with its ensuing imbalance in expenditures, is producing an excessive financial burden on the total population and especially on the poorest groups. Indeed, as a proportion of family income, poor households have higher out-of-pocket expenditures than rich ones. For example, in 1992 the poorest ten per cent of Mexican urban families spent 5.2 per cent of income on healthcare, compared to 2.8 per cent among the richest decile.[10] Two extreme cases are Colombia and Ecuador. Out-of-pocket expenditures for healthcare among the poorest decile of the income distribution reached 12 per cent of household income in Colombia in 1992 and 17 per cent in Ecuador in 1994.

The reasons for the juxtaposition of challenges in the health systems of Latin America are varied. Their roots can be found in the particular historical processes by which economic, political and cultural forces shaped present institutions. A thorough review of such historical factors is beyond the scope of this chapter. Their net result has been the coexistence in the region of several models for organising the financing and delivery of health services. These various models will be described and compared below. Despite their differences, they are all facing serious obstacles to optimal performance.

Indeed, the challenges on both the population and the institutional sides underscore the limitations of the current arrangements for healthcare. In most countries, such arrangements are several decades old. While they may

---

[8] Londoño (1995a).
[9] Fuenzalida-Puelma and Scholle-Connor (1989).
[10] Frenk, Lozano, González Block et al. (1994).

have responded to the conditions prevailing when they were established, health systems have failed to keep pace with the rapid transformation of the epidemiological, demographic, economic, political, technological and cultural context. It is time to devise and test new models for reforming health systems.

Components and functions of health systems

The first step in comparing present arrangements and in designing options for reform is to have a clear conceptualisation about the health system. All too often, health systems are seen as a simple collection of organisations. Instead, we would like to propose a dynamic view of health systems as a set of *structured relationships* among two major components: populations and institutions. It is beyond the scope of this chapter to specify in detail the various dimensions of each of these components.[11] For our present purposes, the important notion is that the various population groups present a series of conditions that constitute health needs requiring an *organised social response* from institutions. In every health system this response is structured through a number of basic functions, which institutions have to perform in order to address the health needs of populations. This notion is schematised in Figure 2.2.

Figure 2.2: Components of Health Systems

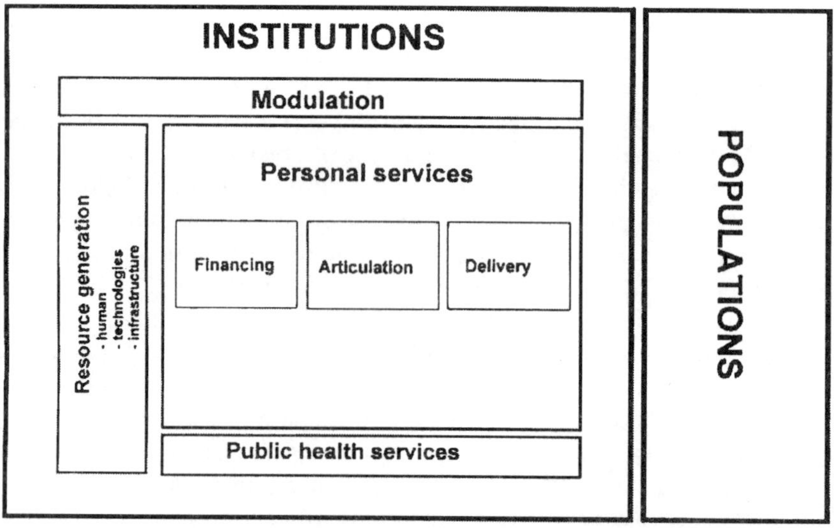

In specifying the functions of the health system, it is useful to bear in mind the conventional distinction between personal and public health services. Most of the discussion that follows will concentrate on personal health serv-

---

[11] The relational view of health systems is explained in greater detail in Frenk (1994).

ices, i.e., the set of preventive, diagnostic, therapeutic and rehabilitative actions that are applied directly to individuals. This emphasis is justified by the fact that personal health services absorb the vast majority of resources and that most of the debates on health system reform refer centrally to them.

Nevertheless, a comprehensive analysis must also include public health services. In the conventional sense, these refer to actions that are applied by health sector agencies either to collectivities (for example, mass health education) or to the non-human components of the environment (for example, basic sanitation). In its modern conception,[12] public health goes beyond those actions that fall within the domain of the health sector narrowly defined, in order to include the interaction with all the other sectors that influence the health of populations. This interaction is a crucial function of any health system.

Figure 2.2 shows another key function: resource generation or production.[13] Indeed, modern health systems are not limited to the set of institutions that provide services, but embrace a diversified group of organisations that produce the inputs to those services. Salient among these are universities and similar institutions, which often have the dual role of developing human resources and providing health services. Another group of important resource generators is made up of research centres producing knowledge and developing new technologies, as well as the large group of firms forming the 'medical-industrial complex', such as pharmaceutical and medical equipment companies.

Although parts of the discussion that follows will also be relevant to public health and to resource generation, the remainder of this chapter will focus, as mentioned above, on personal health services. In this domain, four functions are crucial: modulation, financing, articulation and delivery.[14]

The functions of financing and delivery are the most familiar ones. In its strict sense, financing refers to the mobilisation of money from primary sources (households and firms), as well as from secondary sources (government at all levels and international donors), and its accumulation in real or virtual funds (for example, social insurance funds, public budgets for healthcare, family savings) that can then be allocated through a variety of institutional arrangements to produce services. In turn, the delivery function refers to the combination of inputs into a production process that takes place in a particular organisational structure and that leads to a set of outputs (i.e., health services) which generate an outcome (i.e., changes in the health status of the consumer). As we will discuss later, it is possible to conceive of a 'financing-delivery process' formed by a series of steps or subfunctions. An important aspect

---

[12] Ashton and Seymour (1988); and Frenk (1993).

[13] See Roemer (1991).

[14] Strictly speaking, these four functions also apply to the production of public health services and to resource generation, but our discussion will centre on their implications for the production of personal health services.

of the design of reform options is the distribution of responsibilities for each component of that process.

Alongside the two traditional functions, every health system has to perform a series of key functions, which can be encompassed under the term 'modulation'.[15] This is a broader concept than regulation. It involves setting, implementing and monitoring the rules of the game for the health system, as well as providing it with strategic direction. Setting the rules of the game is a delicate process where the interests of the various actors have to be balanced. Too often, this function has been neglected, particularly in those health systems in which the Ministry of Health devotes most of its human, financial and political resources to the direct delivery of services. Later on, when we propose a new model for health systems, we will argue that modulation must be greatly strengthened. At that point, we will analyse in greater detail the various elements of this key function.

The last function of the health system, as shown in Figure 2.2, can be termed 'articulation'. This function lies between financing and delivery. In most current health systems it has been collapsed into either of those two other functions and has therefore remained implicit. One of the important innovations in many reform proposals has been to make this function explicit and to assign responsibility for performing it to distinct entities. Thus, 'articulation' corresponds to what Chernichovsky calls 'organisation and management of care consumption'.[16] It also encompasses the functions of demand aggregation and consumer representation that are assigned to what the managed competition model calls the 'sponsor'.[17]

The term 'articulation' is meant to convey the notion that this function pulls together and gives coherence to various components of healthcare. As in the case of modulation, we will explain articulation in greater detail later on, when we develop our proposals. At this point it is sufficient to note that articulation encompasses key activities that allow financial resources to flow to the production and consumption of healthcare. Examples include the enrolment of populations into health plans, the specification of explicit packages of benefits or interventions, the organisation of networks of providers so as to structure consumer choices, the design and implementation of incentives to providers through payment mechanisms and the management of quality of care.

The configuration of the four major health system functions — modulation, financing, articulation and delivery — provides the basis to identify the main institutional models. It should be stressed that in some models one or more of the functions may not be explicitly assigned. This is the case of vertically integrated systems, where some functions may be only implicitly performed or may be absent because they conflict with other functions.

---

[15] We are indebted to Professor Avedis Donabedian, from the University of Michigan, for having suggested this term.

[16] Chernichovsky (1995).

[17] Enthoven (1988); Starr (1994).

These omissions are particularly common for modulation and articulation, as we will illustrate in the next section of this chapter. Even the implicit nature or the outright absence of a function reveals important aspects of the character of a health system. While in every health system it is clear who is responsible for financing and delivering services, very often no one is clearly responsible for modulation and articulation. This suggests that reforms should pay special attention to these heretofore-neglected functions.

Based on the conception of the health system as the interaction between populations and institutions, the next section will identify the main models that currently exist in Latin America. By comparing their limitations, it will be possible then to examine the options for a reformed health system.

Current health system models

Through a web of economic, political and cultural forces, every Latin American country has developed a unique health system. Without denying this specificity, it is valid to attempt to identify the common patterns that emerge across countries. Such an exercise can only be possible if one focuses on the essential components of health systems, abstracting from the myriad details that make each national situation unique.

As a result of the historical process of most Latin American countries, the crucial issue that health systems have had to solve is the question of integration. Both in the academic literature and in official documents, this term has been used with multiple and sometimes equivocal usages. It is therefore necessary to specify its meaning. In accordance with our conceptual framework, integration refers to each of the two essential components of health systems: populations and institutions. Based on these two dimensions of integration, Figure 2.3 presents a typology of the main health system models in Latin America.

Figure 2.3: Typology of Health Systems in Latin America

INTEGRATION OF POPULATIONS	INTEGRATION OF INSTITUTIONAL FUNCTIONS	
	Vertical integration	**Separation**
Horizontal integration	Unified public model (e.g., Cuba, Costa Rica)	Public contract model (e.g., Brazil)
Segregation	Segmented model (most Latin American countries)	Atomised private model (e.g., Argentina, Paraguay)

With respect to populations, integration means the extent to which different groups are allowed access to every institution in the health system. Although this is a continuum, it is useful to establish a dichotomy. One end of the dichotomy is segregation. As a reflection of the profound inequalities that affect the region, the health systems of many countries segregate different segments of the population into different healthcare institutions. The financial, and even the legal, possibility of moving across segments is usually limited.[18] The other end of the dichotomy is what could be called 'horizontal integration',[19] where all groups in the population have potential access to all institutions. This situation can be achieved under one of two opposite scenarios: either because there is freedom of choice or because there is a single organisation providing services in the country.

With respect to institutions, integration refers to the arrangements for carrying out the functions described in the previous section of this chapter. Because of the traditional weakness of modulation and articulation, the analysis of the degree of integration centres on the functions of financing and delivery. Again, a dichotomy provides a useful simplification. At one end, there is 'vertical integration', meaning that the same institution carries out the different functions. At the other end, there is separation of functions among different institutions.

Relating the two dimensions of integration, as shown in Figure 2.3, produces a typology of the main health system models that have existed in Latin America until the most recent wave of reforms. It should be noted that no country is a pure expression of any of the models. These represent ideal types that serve to compare the main organisational solutions existing until now. Through such a comparison, the limitations of current arrangements can become apparent and new options can be devised.

For analytical purposes, we will first examine the polar cases, represented by the unified public and the private atomised models.

The unified public model

In this case, the state directly finances and provides health services through a single, vertically integrated system. In its extreme variant, which at present occurs only in Cuba, this model achieves horizontal integration of the population at the expense of freedom of choice, since it is illegal to offer services outside the government monopoly. In accordance with the Latin American bureaucratic tradition, this model excludes delivery options under consumer control and limits effective representation of users in the organisation of services. Faced with a mo-

---

[18] Strictly speaking, segregation is always partial, since in all countries the services provided by the Ministry of Health are, in principle, open to the whole population and the financial barriers are usually the lowest in the system. In contrast, the other segments of the health system do exclude certain social groups either through legal restrictions—as in many social security institutions—or through financial barriers—as in the upper end of the private sector. Therefore, the extent of segregation depends on how important the Ministry of Health is as a provider of services.

[19] We are aware of the fact that other authors use 'horizontal integration' to mean the consolidation, within an organisation, of units that have the same level of complexity or perform the same functions. In our usage, 'horizontal integration' is not a process occurring on the supply (or institutional) side, but on the demand (or population) side of the health system.

nopoly, people cannot choose because, in Hirschman's classical formulation, they lack both voice and exit options.[20] In turn, providers cannot compete to deliver better service, since there are no alternatives.

A less extreme variant of this model can be seen in Costa Rica, where the public system is almost universal, yet there is no legal limitation to choose other service options. In this type of case, the virtual public monopoly is mostly due to the capacity of the government to offer services of a reasonable quality, while competing with the private sector on the basis of price.[21] Since the government does not finance other providers, these must charge what services cost or find a private subsidy. In contrast, public services seldom charge users the real cost. This absence of public subsidy to private provision of services is one of the main features distinguishing the unified public model from the public contract model.[22] In turn, a major difference with respect to the segmented model is that the unified public model maintains one public budget, while in the segmented model public monies are divided between the Ministry of Health and the social security institutions.

In all variants of the unified public model, the modulation function is frequently curtailed by conflicts of interest or because the public monopoly simply does not see the need for this function. For example, when the Ministry of Health is directly involved in the delivery of services, it may be reluctant to promote hospital accreditation for fear that its own facilities would be found deficient. At any rate, modulation is carried out through authoritarian command-and-control modes of operation, which eschew incentives to good performance on the part of providers. In addition, the articulation function is implicit, since vertical integration and lack of competition make it unnecessary to create explicit instances that mediate between financing agencies, providers of care and consumers.

The atomised private model

In this model, the financing function is performed either by out-of-pocket payments from consumers or by many private insurance agencies, which reimburse multiple providers without vertical integration of these two functions. While no Latin American country presents this extreme model in its pure form, there are two important variants that come close to it.

The first one is a free market modality, occurring in countries where the overwhelming majority of expenditures are private and take place in a highly unregulated service delivery environment with low levels of insurance or prepayment. An example is Paraguay, where 87.5 per cent of health expenditures are private.[23] Even though formally there is freedom of choice, the enormous differences in financial accessibility generate an extremely segmented private market, which excludes the majority

---

[20] Hirschman (1970).
[21] Musgrove (1996).
[22] Organisation for Economic Cooperation and Development (OECD, 1992).
[23] Govindaraj, Murray and Chellaraj (1994).

of the population from its upper end. As in the unified public model, in this variant there is no articulation function. In light of the well known imperfections of the market for health services, the diversity of financing and delivery entities does not necessarily produce competition. In fact, the absence of an explicit articulation function means that there is no ready mechanism to aggregate demand, so that consumers can be left unprotected as a result of information asymmetries. Even when there is competition, it often occurs through risk selection rather than through differences in costs or quality. In sum, by excluding large groups of people in need and segmenting the supply of services, market failures generate global inefficiencies in the health system.

The second variant of the atomised private model could be called the 'corporatist' modality.[24] It is characterised by the segregation of different occupational groups into exclusive, non-competitive sickness funds. Although occasionally some funds may have their own delivery facilities, the most common arrangement involves a separation of financing and delivery, so that the sickness funds pay for care that is provided in public or private institutions. This variant is quite infrequent in Latin America. Its exemplar is represented by the system of '*obras sociales*' in Argentina. In contrast to the experience of most of the rest of Latin America, these atomised funds failed to coalesce into a single social security institute. Despite their large number, they do not compete with each other, since there is compulsory affiliation mostly on occupational criteria. The interesting aspect is that these organisations begin to perform the role of articulators, since they aggregate the demands of their affiliates and act as collective purchasers of services.

The public contract model

In a few cases, public financing has been combined with a growing private participation in the delivery of services. This separation of functions is achieved by contracting services. When public financing has universal coverage, horizontal integration of the population is achieved. In Latin America the exemplar of this model has been Brazil in the last decade.

Compared to the polar models, the population increases its options under the public contract model, while providers find more opportunities for autonomy and competition. Usually there is a global public budget, just like in the unified public model. The difference is that the budget is not assigned in advance to public providers regardless of their performance, but is directed to a pluralistic set of providers as a function of certain criteria that reflect productivity and, in the best cases, also quality.

These advantages notwithstanding, a major problem is the lack of an explicit articulation function, which is often collapsed with the financing function. Such deficiency leads to the fragmentation of delivery and

---

[24] We adopt this term from its usage in political science, where corporatism is defined as a system of interest representation characterised by hierarchical and non-competitive occupational associations, which represent their members' interests through direct negotiations with the state. For the classic treatment of this topic, see Schmitter (1979).

makes control of costs and quality extremely cumbersome. The traditional weakness of the modulation function further contributes to the fragmentation of delivery. Although this model resembles some aspects of the Canadian experience, it has lacked its effective modulatory action, which in Canada is greatly strengthened by professional self-regulation. Hence, it has proved impossible for the Latin American version to achieve the levels of equity and efficiency of the Canadian health system.

The segmented model

This is the most common model in Latin America. Its structure can be depicted in a simplified way with the matrix shown in Figure 2.4a. This matrix relates the health system functions described earlier with the various social groups.[25] Typically, health systems in Latin America have been divided into three segments, each designed to serve a social group.

Figure 2.4a: Present Design of the Segmented Model

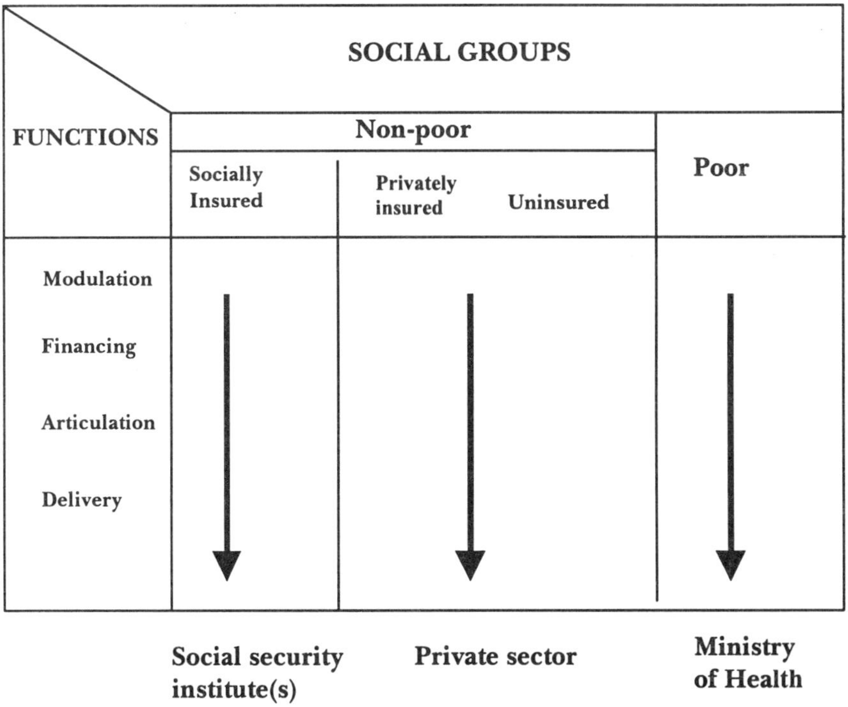

FUNCTIONS	SOCIAL GROUPS			
	Non-poor			Poor
	Socially Insured	Privately insured	Uninsured	
Modulation				
Financing				
Articulation				
Delivery				
	Social security institute(s)	Private sector		Ministry of Health

An initial fundamental distinction has been made between the poor and the non-poor. In turn, the latter comprise two groups. The first one is formed

---

[25] Frenk, Lozano, González Block et al. (1994).

by those working in the formal sector of the economy (and often their relatives as well), who are covered by one or several social security institutes.

The second group comprises the middle and upper classes, mostly urban, which are not protected by social security.[26] The health needs of this group are mostly catered to by the private sector, with financing coming principally from out-of-pocket payments. Increasingly, some middle and upper class families get coverage from private insurance or prepaid plans, whether purchased directly or offered through employers. While this is still a minority option in the overall picture of the region, in many countries it is expanding rapidly. At any rate, these forms of private insurance fit in the general model as one more modality of private involvement.

Finally, there are the poor, both rural and urban, who are excluded from social security because they do not have formal employment. In the design of the segmented model, ministries of health are charged with providing personal health services to the poor (in addition, of course, to carrying out public health programmes that benefit the whole population).

On average for Latin America, approximately one-third of the population is affiliated to a social security institute, one third receives most of its care from public-sector facilities and another third goes mostly to the private sector.[27]

As can be seen in Figure 2.4a, the segmented model segregates the three population groups into their respective institutional niches. Indeed, this model can be described as a system of vertical integration but horizontal segregation. Each institutional segment — the Ministry of Health, the social security institutes and the private sector — performs the functions of modulation, financing, articulation (when present) and delivery of services, but does so only for a specific group.

Such a configuration of the health system has many problems. First, it makes for duplication and waste of resources, especially in high-technology services. Second, it usually leads to major quality differentials among the various segments. In particular, services reserved for the poor suffer from a chronic shortage of resources.[28] Third, segmentation actually implies the coexistence of the two polar models and combines the disadvantages of the two. Thus, the integrated Ministry of Health has all the shortcomings of the unified public model, but without the advantage of universal coverage. Similarly, each social security institution exercises a monopoly over its respective clientele. And the private sector presents all the limitations that were discussed earlier for the atomised private model. Most of these deficiencies are due not so much to the existence of the three segments per se, but to the hermetic vertical integration within each

---

[26] Strictly speaking, many members of these classes, especially those with higher incomes, do pay social security contributions, but they never use its services. In actual fact, these persons see their contributions to social security as one more tax, rather than as an insurance premium.

[27] These figures were derived from country-level estimates produced by the Pan American Health Organisation (PAHO, 1994).

[28] Musgrove (1996).

one. Paradoxically, this segmentation creates incentives for many health professionals (mostly physicians) to seek employment in more than one institution, typically by combining a salaried job in a public organisation with private practice. Such a combination often creates conflicts of interest (for example, patients being referred from the public organisation to the private practice) and leads to differentials in the quality standards applied by the same physician, which are very problematic from the point of view of professional ethics and of social justice.

While all the aforementioned limitations are serious, the most important problem with the design of the segmented model is that it does not reflect actual population behaviour. Indeed, people do not necessarily respect the artificial divisions among the three segments. In fact, there is a considerable overlap of demand, with a very high proportion of social-security beneficiaries using services provided by the private sector or the Ministry of Health.[29] The problem is that the burden of such a decision is borne by the consumer, for he or she is forced to pay for the care received elsewhere, despite already having paid an insurance premium. This leads to an important source of inequity: multiple payments, which impose on many families and businesses a disproportionate financial burden.

Another source of inequity is that the overlap in demand is unilateral, since uninsured families cannot use social-security facilities (except in emergencies and a few high-priority services). Furthermore, many ministries of health have failed in their intended targeting of services for the poor. The notion that private services are reserved to the middle and upper classes, thereby liberating public resources to care for the poor, is not supported by utilisation data. In most countries with such data, it turns out that the private sector is an important source of care for poor households, which spend a much higher proportion of their income on out-of-pocket payments than richer households, as was demonstrated earlier.

The search for new options

The many shortcomings of the four models analysed so far has led to an intensive search for other solutions, which has inspired the health system reform movement in Latin America and other parts of the world.

In particular, the most common current arrangement, represented by the segmented model, has increasingly been brought under scrutiny. Because this model segregates population groups with different abilities to pay and social organisation, its sustainability depends on the duality of labour markets and on exclusionary state policies. With economic modernisation and the expansion of democracy, the privileges entailed by this model for relatively small groups have been increasingly difficult to sustain. Therefore, there have been numerous efforts to correct the failures of segmented systems. So far, these efforts have gone in two directions. Interestingly, they point towards the polar models.

---

[29] González-Block (1994).

Some countries have attempted to break the segmentation of the population by nationalising the health services and unifying all institutions in a single public system. This was probably the most popular reform strategy up until the 1980s and still has many proponents. The search for equity under this strategy has proved to be incompatible with the requirements of efficiency and responsiveness to populations' needs and preferences.

Either because of ideological preferences or public finance restrictions, other countries have sought to hand over the organisation of health services to entities other than the central government. In Latin America there have been two variants of this type of reform. The first has been the privatisation strategy, particularly with respect to social security. The ISAPREs in Chile are the best example of the policy to give greater weight to the private sector. The second variant has been the decentralisation strategy, with devolution of previously centralised responsibilities to local authorities. Brazil and Bolivia are noteworthy examples. A major problem with both variants has been the weakness of the modulatory effort needed to set clear rules of the game for the transfer of responsibilities. Instead, central decision-makers have acted under the implicit assumption that local or private initiative will somehow solve the major limitations in healthcare. Under these conditions, many privatisation and decentralisation initiatives have proved to be incompatible with the requirements of equity and, paradoxically, have not yielded the expected gains in efficiency.

As can be seen, there are serious drawbacks to those reform strategies that have simply moved within the limited options offered by the four conventional models. Because of this, a growing number of countries have started to look for truly innovative alternatives. In this context of innovation, several proposed and implemented reform initiatives have started to develop an option that seeks to minimise the disadvantages and optimise the advantages of the other models, so as to achieve an optimal balance among equity, efficiency and quality. While the existing proposals and experiences show important differences, this emerging model is well captured with the term 'structured pluralism'. We next describe this promising alternative.

An innovative model: structured pluralism

The concept of 'structured pluralism' tries to convey the search for a middle ground between the extreme arrangements that have so much hampered the performance of health systems. 'Pluralism' avoids the extremes of monopoly in the public sector and atomisation in the private sector. 'Structured' avoids the extremes of authoritarian command-and-control procedures in government and the anarchic absence of transparent rules of the game to correct market failures. In this respect, it is interesting to note that opposite extremes can end up having the same deleterious effect. For example, subordination of consumers to providers and insurers is a common outcome of both the unified public model — through lack of choice — and the atomised private model — through information asymmetry. Very often the real dilemma is not between public or private ownership of facilities, but between provider, insurer or consumer sovereignty. Structured pluralism fosters a more balanced distribution of power than either of the polar models has achieved.

Just as the segmented model mixes the disadvantages of these extreme models, so structured pluralism compensates for them. This solution can be visualised by referring back to the matrix of functions and social groups. As shown in Figure 2.4b, the proposal is to turn the matrix around. Instead of the present vertical integration with segregation of social groups, there would be horizontal integration of the population with explicit and specialised assignment of functions. In other words, the health system would no longer be organised by social groups, but by functions.[30] Indeed, a key feature of this model is that it identifies explicitly each of the four functions. In this way, it promotes a specialisation of actors in the health system. This is why structured pluralism involves a new institutional configuration for the health system.

Figure 2.4b: Proposed Design of Structured Pluralism

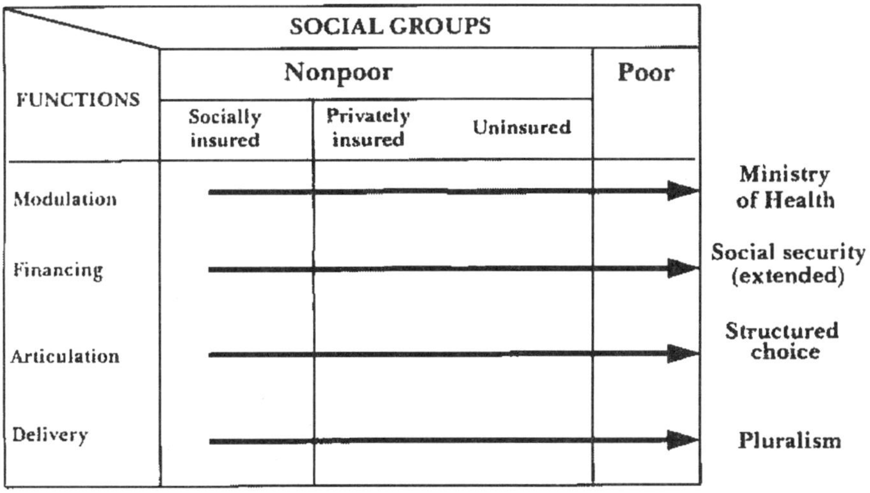

In this scheme, modulation would become the main mission of the Ministry of Health, as the entity in charge of giving strategic direction to the whole system. Instead of being one more provider of services — usually the weakest — the Ministry of Health would assure a balanced, efficient and equitable interaction among all actors by structuring the appropriate rules and incentives. As will be argued below, this emphasis on modulation should not lead to bu-

---

[30] Frenk, Lozano, González Block et al. (1994).

reaucratic concentration of power. On the contrary, having set transparent and fair rules of the game, ministries of health could increasingly delegate the actual operation of many modulatory functions to participatory organisations of civil society that are not captured by special interests.

The next function, financing, would become the major responsibility of social security, which would be gradually extended in order to achieve universal protection under principles of public finance. Compared with current financial arrangements, there would be a greater emphasis on demand-side than on supply-side subsidies. Instead of allocating a historical budget to each facility regardless of performance, each insured person would represent a potential payment contingent on the choice of insurer and provider by the consumer.

Managing that payment would be a key element of the articulation function, which would now become explicit and would be carried out by specialised institutions. These could generically be called 'organisations for health services articulation' (OHSAs). As will be explained later on, there are several options for the specific development of these organisations, depending on the conditions of each country. In urban areas, these organisations would compete to enrol individuals and families. In rural areas, conditions are usually not ready for this kind of open competition. Nevertheless, even there it is possible to foster pluralism that is responsive to population needs. Indeed, in order to stimulate choice and efficiency it is not necessary to have all the conditions for full-blown competition. Often, it suffices to have 'market contestability', which refers to the potential participation of alternative agencies for the organisation of services, in a situation where block grants or annual contracts can only be arranged with one such agency. For many rural areas in Latin America, market contestability would be obtained if several agencies would compete annually for broad contracts to serve specific populations. Some innovations already point to such possibilities, like the cooperatives organised in Colombia as 'solidarity health enterprises' and the type of franchises proposed for Mexico.[31]

Finally, as a consequence of greater choice in the articulation function, the direct delivery of services would be opened up to a pluralistic array of institutions, both public and private.

In sum, the challenge for structured pluralism is to increase the options both for consumers and for providers, while having explicit rules of the game that will minimise the potential conflicts between equity and efficiency. An increase in the options for consumers is accompanied by an extension of prepayment in a context of public finance to assure and redistribute resources. An increase in the options for providers is accompanied by their integration into efficient networks, which are clearly articulated and modulated.

In terms of our original typology of health system models in Latin America, structured pluralism adopts the positive aspects of the public contract model, while overcoming its limitations. Mobility of the popula-

---

[31] *Ibid.*

tion through horizontal integration is preserved, as is the separation of functions. The major difference from the public contract model is that the modulation and articulation functions are made explicit and greatly strengthened. Alongside the traditional functions of financing and delivery, it is the emphasis on modulation and articulation what gives the 'structured' character to this kind of pluralism.

Given the centrality of these two functions, it is necessary to explain them in greater detail.

Modulation: the neglected function

There seems to be a growing awareness that the modulation function has been insufficiently specified and implemented in most health systems. As these systems become more open and diverse through decentralisation and increased competition, modulation will have to be strengthened. This is a key feature for present and future reforms.

Increasingly, discussions about reform options are focusing on the need to establish fair and transparent rules of the game, in order to foster a harmonious development of the system. Such rules are the essence of institutions, as they make it possible to reduce uncertainty by providing stability to interactions.[32] This is a specialised function that must be differentiated from both financing and delivery, so as to avoid conflicts of interest and assure the transparency of the myriad transactions occurring in modern health systems. Hence, modulation must be carried out by neutral instances that can rise above any special interest.

While there is still much to be debated and decided concerning the specifics of modulation, in practically all health systems this function is a public responsibility. This does not mean that the actual *operation* of all modulatory functions must be carried out by the government. In fact, there is cross-national variation in the extent to which other actors participate in the operation of some of those functions (like certification or accreditation). Nonetheless, there is widespread consensus that the ultimate *responsibility* is public, meaning that a politically legitimate agent must be responsive and accountable to the interests of the entire collectivity. As explained below, in almost all countries modulation encompasses a core of public functions.

In contrast, there is wide variation in the degree of state intervention concerning the other three functions of the health system (i.e., financing, articulation and delivery). The real debate no longer concerns a Manichæan choice between statisation or privatisation, but the best distribution of functions between public and private institutions so as to optimise population wellbeing. In this public/private mix, the importance of modulation as an essential public responsibility is underscored precisely by the growing pluralism in the other functions.

---

[32] North (1990).

In fact, the emphasis on modulation represents a shift in the conception about the central mission of ministries of health. It is therefore part of the broader discussion about the reform of the state that has been going on in Latin America. This reform has proposed that public organisations should stop being owners of facilities and producers of goods and services. Instead, government should channel its energy into promoting public interest; proposing strategic directions; providing comprehensive security; mobilising resources; setting standards; catalysing private activity; giving transparency to markets; protecting consumers; evaluating performance and assuring justice.

When translated to the specific realm of healthcare, the reform of the state means that ministries of health should gradually move away from the direct provision of services, into the strategic modulation of the system. Of course, government retains a direct responsibility for the financing and delivery of those health services that have the characteristics of public goods, such as epidemiological surveillance and environmental sanitation. Even in this case, however, there are many possible innovations for governments to fulfil their responsibility through efficient, responsive, participatory and autonomous modes of organisation.

Shifting their central mission towards modulation would actually strengthen ministries of health. It is the concern with the details of direct operation of services that weakens ministries of health. Their true strength lies in their capacity to mobilise social energy for a common purpose. Such a catalytic role is the essence of modulation. In order to perform it, modulation includes five more specific functions:

1. **System development:** in turn, this includes the following elements:

- Policy formulation

- Strategic planning

- Priority setting for resource allocation, including the process of building consensus around those priorities

- Intersectoral advocacy, so as to promote 'healthy policies' that will act on the social, economic, environmental and cultural determinants of health status

- Social mobilisation for health, including community participation

- Development of criteria and standards for the assessment of performance of financing agencies, articulating organisations and individual and institutional providers of services

- Capacity strengthening through promotion of investments in physical infrastructure, human resources, scientific research, technological development and information systems

2. **Coordination:** there are many situations in healthcare that require concerted action in order to achieve objectives efficiently. This is the case, for example, of complex and costly tertiary technologies where it may be desirable to limit the number of providers in order to achieve economies of scale. Another case is represented by massive public health campaigns, which commonly involve the collaboration of many organisations. In general, coordination may be required among territorial units, levels of government, or public and private organisations. There must be an instance in the health system with the authority to convene these multiple actors in the pursuit of common objectives.

This does not mean, however, that coordination must be carried out in an authoritarian manner. On the contrary, one of the challenges for new institutional development under structured pluralism involves the promotion of efficient and equitable modalities of transaction among public and private agents. The task of coordination becomes then one of strategic design that will give transparency and consistency to those transactions. Hence, coordination should not be carried out through discretionary interventions by bureaucracies, but through clear rules of the game that facilitate interactions in a pluralistic environment. Once those rules are set as a part of modulation, the actual activities leading to coordination of healthcare can then be performed as part of the articulation function, as will be explained below. For example, contracts and information represent valuable tools to achieve transparent coordination in healthcare. A system increasingly based on explicit contracts for the performance of functions can produce a more efficient and less authoritarian control of compliance. The provision of information so that every actor can make rational decisions and the others can know about them is another essential element of this new institutional development.

3. **Financial design:** in order to increase coverage and quality, modern health systems must face two key financial challenges: to mobilise the required resources and contain costs. Often, progress on one of these fronts can create obstacles for the other. Hence, it is necessary to strike a balance between both. Such a balance can only be achieved through a careful design of the financial scheme. The design of financing, as distinct from its operation, is an important part of modulation. Without a careful design, the system can suffer either from shortage of resources or from cost explosion. Setting clear financial rules is essential to achieve a sustainable reform. In particular, this part of modulation aims at providing global consistency to the resources in the system — something that has been absent in the segmented, the atomised and the public contract models. Without such financial consistency there can be no rationality.

The function of financial design involves key decisions that will determine the structure of incentives in the system, such as the use of public funds for the benefit packages (especially if they are mandated); the amounts of capitation payments and the possible risk adjustments for them; the budget cap for the system as a whole; the formulas for re-source allocation among territorial units, levels of government or non-governmental institutions; and the use of policy instruments, like taxes and subsidies, that are aimed at changing population behaviour.

4. **Regulation strictly speaking:** This includes two main types: sanitary regulation of goods and services and healthcare regulation. The former refers to the conventional efforts by health authorities to minimise the health hazards that might be generated by the goods and services pro-vided throughout the economy, especially those that are directly con-sumed by human beings, such as foodstuffs.

Even more crucial to our present discussion is the second kind of regulation, which is applied to the specific sectors of the economy deal-ing directly with healthcare. Thus, this type of regulation is designed to set rules for the following components of the health system:

- Individual providers, through licensure and certification

- Institutional providers, through accreditation

- Financing mechanisms, through rules for insurance funds and similar instruments

- Organisations in charge of the articulation function, through ac-creditation and supervision, so as to ensure their accountability to consumers, as discussed below

- Educational institutions, through accreditation

- Drugs, equipment and devices, through technology assessment

- Capital investments, through plans

These regulatory activities must be carried out in a decentralised man-ner and with the active participation of all actors. In fact, the operation of many regulatory procedures can be delegated to organisations of civil society, with the appropriate safeguards so that the regulatory process is not captured by special interests. The final aim must be to create struc-tural conditions for improving the quality of healthcare.

5. **Consumer protection:** The important information asymmetry that characterises the healthcare market makes it necessary to have an explicit strategy for consumer protection. A first instrument in this respect is to offer public information about the performance of insurers and providers. Mak-ing this kind of information available to consumers and to OHSAs (as agents in the purchase of health services) would foster effective competition.

Of course, the mere dissemination of information is not enough to redress fully the power imbalance among providers and consumers. It is also necessary to develop a deliberate effort — until now very much ne-glected — for human rights protection and conflict mediation.

In sum, the type of modulation that structured pluralism calls for does not create obstacles to the market for health services, but is instead a necessary condition for it to function in a transparent and efficient manner. The function of articulation is also crucial to this purpose.

Articulation: the innovative function

In order to understand this concept better, it is useful to think in terms of a 'financing-delivery process', that is to say, a continuum of activities whereby financial resources are mobilised and allocated in order to make possible the production and consumption of health services. The first step in this process is the actual collection of money from the population by financing agencies and the accumulation of that money into funds. Organised in households and in firms, the population represents the ultimate financial source, through general taxes, payroll and other earmarked contributions and premiums. Once the members of a population have transferred resources to financing agencies, there are two major interfaces that must be articulated in parallel: on the one hand, between populations and providers; on the other, between financing agencies and providers.

1. **Articulation between populations and providers**: This part of the articulation function includes at least three major subfunctions: risk management, access management and representation.

Risk management is performed by enrolling populations so that risks are spread, thereby reducing the financial uncertainty of consumers in their interaction with providers. OHSAs receive payment in exchange for assuming the risks entailed in covering uncertain events. To establish an expenditure cap, while at the same time creating an equitable incentive against competition on the basis of risk selection, such payment should be a risk-adjusted capitation.

However, articulation goes a step beyond the traditional insurance function, since it also encompasses access management. This subfunction operationalises several crucial aspects of the interaction between populations and providers, including the procedures for entry and exit by clients into and from the health system; the set of contingencies to be covered, defined through an explicit package of benefits or interventions (often publicly mandated); and the range of choices available to consumers, structured through the organisation of comprehensive networks of providers.

Finally, the articulating organisation acts as the informed agent of consumers and represents their aggregate interests (as well as those of the financing agency) by serving as a prudent purchaser of health services on their behalf.

Through these three subfunctions it is possible to match the heterogeneous demands of consumers with the complex and specialised capacities of providers so as to assure cost-effective use of resources, good technical quality and user satisfaction. It is this explicit articulation of resources, providers and consumers that constitutes one of the innovations proposed by structured pluralism.

2. **Articulation between financing agencies and providers**: Articulation mediates between financial agencies and providers by selectively channelling the resources of the former into the latter. It does so through three subfunctions: incentive design, benefit design and quality management. The key aspect of incentive design is the payment mechanism. If properly structured, the way providers are paid can foster their efficiency and their responsiveness to consumers. Another crucial aspect of system design refers to the package of benefits or interventions.[33] Through adequate benefit design, the financing agency can be assured that its resources are being applied in the most cost-effective manner, so that it gets the best value for money. Finally, the articulating organisation can perform important functions for the management of quality, such as certifying the competence of providers and monitoring the processes and outcomes of care, including both its technical aspects and consumer satisfaction.

As can be seen, the articulation function allows for a transparent connection among the various components of the financing-delivery process. The search for this transparency has been a common feature of several reform initiatives. In many of the recent European proposals, one way of articulating those components has been through contracts among the financial agencies, the providers of services and the consumers. OHSAs represent a similar but more structured modality, which links users to global financing, while organising comprehensive networks of providers. One of the main advantages of this proposal is that it fosters a simplification of public tasks, since it replaces bureaucratic control for direct interrelationships among actors based on appropriate incentives.

In this way, new forms of linkage are developed which go beyond the simple separation of financing and delivery so current in the literature. Functionally, the separation between financing and delivery is maintained at the level of health system. Organisationally, the articulating entities can carry out several of the functions in the financing-delivery process, as they seek the most efficient forms of integration. As mentioned earlier, OHSAs can thereby go beyond the classical insurance function and play a more active role in the healthcare market as purchasing agents in the name of consumers. Instead of being passive *payers* like traditional insurance companies, they become active *purchasers* of services. In this way, OHSAs can guarantee, for a predefined population, access to a package of interventions. In order to do so, they organise different types of providers on the basis of incentives designed to improve efficiency and responsiveness to clients. At the same time, OHSAs act on behalf of consumers so that they can exercise greater freedom of choice in the search for continuity and quality of care.

---

[33] Jamison, Mosley, Measham and Bobadilla (eds.) (1993).

In Latin America there is a growing presence of organisations that are performing some or all aspects of articulation. These include the Empresas Promotoras de Salud (EPSs) in Colombia, the Instituciones de Atención Médica Colectiva (IAMCs) in Uruguay, the *obras sociales* in Argentina, many of the *prepagadas* in Brazil, the *igualas* in the Dominican Republic, many of the Instituciones de Salud Previsional (ISAPREs) in Chile and the proposed Organizaciones para la Protección de la Salud (PROSALUD) in Mexico. The magnitude of this emerging phenomenon is considerable. We estimate that these organisations cover at present more than 60 million Latin Americans. Their performance varies widely. Some of them continue to function simply as traditional insurers. Others are approaching the ideal of a fully developed OHSA. Performance seems to be less effective when these organisations operate under either of two extremes: unregulated competition or absence of competition. Structuring competition through modulation and articulation offers a balanced middle point between these two extremes, with the potential for important improvements in the performance of health systems.

Towards institutional convergence in Latin America

The expansion of innovative experiences in Latin America is already putting in place some of the building blocks of structured pluralism. Furthermore, many current reform proposals also point in that direction. An interesting characteristic of structured pluralism is that it is possible to move towards it through different paths. To illustrate this notion, Figure 2.5 arranges the health system models in terms of the way in which they have solved the linkages among modulation (or only regulation), financing, articulation and delivery. The multiple bars in the segmented and the atomised public models represent the fact that different population groups are segregated into different institutional arrangements. The different letter types for modulation/regulation and articulation are meant to illustrate the fact that these functions become more explicit and important as one moves toward the middle model of structured pluralism.

In the case of the unified public model, it would be necessary to transform bureaucratic regulation into real modulation, separate financing from delivery and make the articulation function explicit. In the other polar model (i.e., atomised private), it would also be necessary to modulate the operation of the insurance and services markets, while establishing OHSAs, which would compete in order to make freedom of choice a reality for all the population. Increasing population mobility would also be a priority in the segmented model, which would be achieved by separating functions and competitively opening up each segment. The public contract model would require the articulation function to be made explicit and competitive by separating it from financing. In addition, all the existing models would require a strengthening of modulation, as described earlier.

Figure 2.5: Convergence among Health System Models

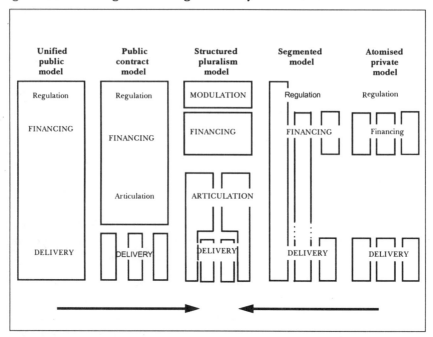

The key message is that structured pluralism does not offer a single path for reform. What it does offer is a 'centrist' option, which avoids extremes, while allowing a dynamic convergence from all starting points. In so doing, structured pluralism pays careful attention to establishing the necessary checks and balances among the various actors in the system. Thus, OHSAs have to manage a delicate equilibrium between the incentives to cost-containment implicit in capitation payments and the imperative to satisfy consumers promoted by freedom of choice. Equity is pursued by public finance principles, by eliminating segregation barriers and by deterring competition on the basis of risk selection. At the same time, fairness in remuneration is advanced by risk-adjusting capitation payments and by recognising superior performance. It is this balanced pursuit of equity, quality and efficiency that has eluded existing models and that structured pluralism explicitly tries to achieve.

The innovative experiences already underway and the converging elements present in most reform proposals provide grounds for optimism. Yet, with the notable exception of the recent reform in Colombia, which is developing a comprehensive and universal approach to structured pluralism, and of the interesting efforts in Argentina and Brazil, most of the innovations in Latin America have been restricted to particular population groups, especially urban middle classes. Thus, they run the risk of becoming one more segment in the health system. Even though many of its pieces are already in place, there is still much to be done in order to implement structured pluralism as a comprehensive model. For this to happen, reform initiatives must move structured pluralism beyond the realm of limited innovations and make it the centrepiece of public policy. This would imply a strategy to extend this model gradually to the entire population. To do so, it is necessary to take into account the heterogeneity of populations in each of the countries of Latin America.

Responding to population heterogeneity

Just as structured pluralism does not offer a single path to every country, so it does not present a single approach to every population group within each country. On the contrary, this model is sensitive to the enormous social differences that exist in most Latin American countries. What structured pluralism offers is not a single solution, but rather a *continuum of solutions*, depending on the overall development situation.

The challenge is to offer solutions that are adequate for each group without falling again into the segregation of the segmented model. Structured pluralism meets this challenge in three ways. First, it maintains the same values and principles for all population groups: for example, the search for balanced answers that avoid extremes; the simultaneous emphasis on equity, efficiency and quality; the elaboration of transparent rules of the game through fair modulation; the explicitness of articulation; the importance of information; the plurality of options; the design of as much freedom of choice as possible in each circumstance; the equilibrium of power among all actors; and the systemic approach. Second, structured pluralism avoids segregation by deliberately strengthening the mobility of all social groups among the various institutional solutions. Third, under structured pluralism everyone is protected by insurance, with explicit subsidies for those who cannot afford it, so that the insured/uninsured distinction ceases to exist.

In order to understand the specific way in which the pluralistic model responds to the needs of different populations, it is useful to consider that there are three major social groups in Latin America: a) the extreme poverty core, which is mostly located in dispersed rural areas and periurban slums; b) the informal sectors living in poverty, which are mostly located in urban and periurban areas; c) the formal sectors, which are concentrated in the urban areas. The proportions of these groups vary enormously among the Latin American countries. Every country will therefore adopt the policy prescriptions that are best suited to its levels of heterogeneity. Let us briefly consider the key responses that structured pluralism offers for each of the three populations.

For the extreme poverty core, present access to formal health services is nil or minimal (often limited to sporadic public health campaigns). To correct this situation, a central policy instrument is a package of *essential* interventions. The word 'essential' is key, and it must be sharply differentiated from adjectives like 'minimal' or 'basic'. The essential package is not based on a principle of 'the least for the poor',' but rather on one of 'the best for all'. Indeed, this package is formed by those interventions that cost-effectiveness analysis has shown to be the very best investments for health. They therefore constitute the nucleus of universality, that is to say, the set of interventions that every person, regardless of his or her financial capabilities or labour market situation, must have access to. This new type of universality, which is oriented by explicit cost-effectiveness analysis and social acceptability, avoids the pitfalls of classical universality, whose promise of 'everything for everyone' has proved to be unsustainable even in the wealthiest countries. In this sense, cost-effectiveness analysis is much more than a technocratic tool, since it represents a scientifically based, ethically sound and socially acceptable means of achieving the optimal allocation of resources for health. Hence, an essential package promotes both equity and allocational efficiency. Because it represents a social commitment based on citizenship principles, financing must be mostly public. As pointed out earlier, structured pluralism makes the definition of the essential package a key element of participatory modulation. At the same time, it introduces organisational innovations so that the articulation function can be carried out in a pluralistic framework actively involving the community.

The second social group is formed by those persons who already have partial access to health services, but who are left without financial protection because they form part of the informal sector of the economy and are therefore excluded from social security. Therefore, a major policy prescription is to extend social insurance with an explicit package of benefits, to be financed through prepayment and a demand-side subsidy geared to household income. In order to avoid the pitfalls of traditional social insurance, structured pluralism proposes that, from the beginning, this type of programme be based on clear modulation, explicit articulation and freedom of choice of primary providers so as to start stimulating competitive forces.

The third group is formed by the population in the formal economy, who have access to comprehensive services with financial protection (mostly through social security), although with all the problems of equity, efficiency and quality discussed earlier. In this case, cost-effectiveness analysis comes into play as a tool of technology assessment, which makes it possible to identify wasteful investments and restrict their adoption through modulatory action and incentive design. In addition to this concern with allocational efficiency, the policy process must deal with issues of equity, technical efficiency and quality (including patient satisfaction). For this population conditions are ripe to implement structured competition fully. This is the most developed variant of structured pluralism, where full specialisation of functions among agents can be achieved and where horizontally integrated populations exercising freedom of choice drive competition among articulating entities and providers. The requirements for this form of competition are met in major Latin American cities, where there is generally an abundant supply of providers, the presence of relatively well informed consumers and the necessary levels of institutional development.

For all three population groups, a central feature of structured pluralism is the public character of financing. For the poorest group, this takes the form of direct subsidies. For the two other groups, it takes the form of mandatory contributions, which anticipate disease events. The application of public finance principles differentiates our model from reform proposals simply centred on cost recovery. It also introduces an important difference with respect to several managed competition proposals, since in our model pluralism is concentrated on the articulation and delivery functions and not on financing.

In sum, structured pluralism can respond to the diverse conditions present in a country, while maintaining the mobility of all groups as they converge towards comprehensive coverage with financial protection and freedom of choice.

Towards implementation: instruments and strategies

Progress in the reform agenda is not based only on an accurate diagnosis of current deficiencies and a rigorous design of the preferred model to improve the situation. It is also necessary to move towards questions of implementation, which have two main dimensions: the technical and the political.

Technical dimension: the instruments of reform

The number of useful instruments to improve policy formulation and implementation in health has grown during the past years. Indeed, the analytical and management armamentarium has been enriched by several innovative approaches. While many of them still require adjustments and others still remain to be developed, there is much that the decision-maker can do today. Of course, it would be naïve to assume that decision-makers always base their actions on objective evidence brought about by the application of analytical instruments. Often, such evidence is not available. Even when it is, the decision-maker, particularly in the public sector, must balance the weight of technical recommendations against the political feasibility of following the desired course of action.

While it is clear that decisions are made on the basis of many other forces apart from information, it is also true that good evidence can steer those who have the power to decide into a better course of action. At the very least, effective instruments place limits on the discretion of decision-makers. But such instruments can also empower the decision-maker, who can better counter the vested interests that oppose an enlightened decision. He or she may then be more willing to assume the risks of innovation.[34]

That is why one cannot underestimate the value of good analytical and management instruments to orient health system reform. Their development must therefore be a priority. Before focusing specifically on the instruments available for the implementation of structured pluralism, it is useful to consider that these are part of a broader armamentarium, which includes the following categories:

---

[34] Frenk (1995).

1. **Advocacy instruments:** These make it possible to link the health agenda to broader concerns of economic and social policy (for example, analysis of health contributions to human capital formation and to economic growth).

2. **Diagnostic instruments:** These help to identify and quantify the main challenges facing the policy-maker in two domains: a) the health conditions of the population (for example, burden of disease analysis); and b) the response by institutions (for example, organisational analysis, measurement of performance, political mapping).

3. **Instruments for identification of options**: These facilitate the design and choice of alternative courses of action to improve the health system (for example, cost-effectiveness analysis of interventions, technology assessment, comparative analysis of previous reforms).

4. **Instruments for implementation of solutions**: As stated earlier, our discussion will centre on those instruments that can help to advance the practical adoption of reforms.

Until now, most implementation instruments have focused on the supply (or provider) side and have ignored the demand (or population) side of healthcare. An additional problem is that supply-side instruments have not been sensitive to performance. Conventional instruments include historical budgets, regulations, investment plans and various programming techniques. It is necessary to develop and utilise performance-based instruments that create the appropriate incentives for the supply side. It is also necessary to act on the demand side, so as to achieve the type of comprehensive perspective advocated by structured pluralism.

In an effort to advance this perspective systematically, Figures 2.6a and 2.6b show the main instruments available to implement reform initiatives based on structured pluralism. The instruments are arranged in accordance with our previous conceptual discussion, looking both at the population and at the institutions that perform the different functions. While the titles of most instruments shown in Figures 2.6a and 2.6b are self-explanatory, there is often an active discussion regarding the different variants of each of them. A review of such discussion is beyond the scope of this chapter.

Generally speaking, most of the implementation instruments can be classified in the two categories according to which Figures 2.6a and 2.6b have been divided. Thus, Figure 2.6a shows the main **financial instruments** (for example, prepayment; contributions; subsidies; financial accountability requirements like solvency and liquidity; accounting systems; capitation; risk adjustment; contracts and agreements; copayments and deductibles). In turn, Figure 2.6b presents the main organisational instruments, which can be further grouped into: a) **priority-setting instruments** (for example, benefit packages, cost-effectiveness analysis, technology assessment); b) **quality improvement instruments** (for example, licensure, certification, accreditation, benchmarking, monitoring and assurance of both technical quality and consumer satisfaction); and c) **institutional configuration instruments** (for example, public information, consumer protection, enrolment, consumer choice, access management, provider autonomy).

Figure 2.6a: Main Financial Instruments for Implementing Health System Reform

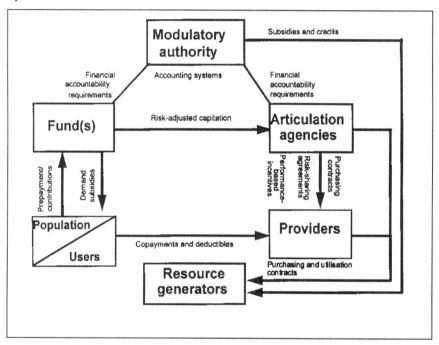

The main purpose of Figures 2.6a and 2.6b is to illustrate the notion that there is a growing body of technical means to put the principles of structured pluralism into practice. A necessary complement to this technical dimension is represented by the political strategies to increase the feasibility of reform.

Political dimension: strategies for feasibility

As we have seen throughout this chapter, the main problems of healthcare in Latin America are systemic. Systems have various components, which can be modified with policy interventions through the use of the instruments mentioned in the previous section. A variety of specific actors participate in the design and execution of such interventions. The key to the success of any reform process will be to match intervention instruments effectively with actors that make their application feasible.

Figure 2.6b: Main Organisational Instruments for Implementing Health System Reform

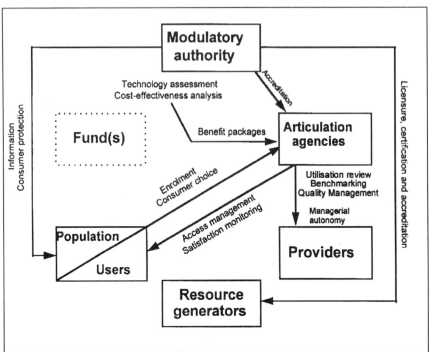

In the long run, reforms will function if the necessary instruments are utilised in a consistent fashion and are accepted by all the actors in the system. Nevertheless, decision-makers usually face serious constraints in terms of time and capacity to coordinate. Hence, the design of a political strategy can be more or less ambitious depending on the combinations of actions and actors. Figure 2.7 presents the possible political strategies by combining two analytical dimensions. One dimension portrays the scope of actions, ranging from partial changes to comprehensive reforms. The other dimension ranges from low to high levels of consensus on the proposed policy interventions. Each of the resulting strategies leads to certain problems.

The major temptation in confronting a systemic problem is to attempt to generate a comprehensive set of policy interventions. Energetic and ambitious authorities often want to accomplish everything during their limited time in office. This decision to adopt a comprehensive scope for policy actions can, in turn, be combined with different degrees of consensus among actors. It is possible, especially in societies with stronger parliamentary traditions, to try to involve society as a whole. In societies with a more executive tradition, it is common to try to implement comprehensive policies investing less effort in the search for consensus. Alternatively, authorities may focus their attention on a more reduced set of policy interventions, searching for higher or lower levels of consensus among actors.

Figure 2.7: Political Strategies for Implementing Health System Reform

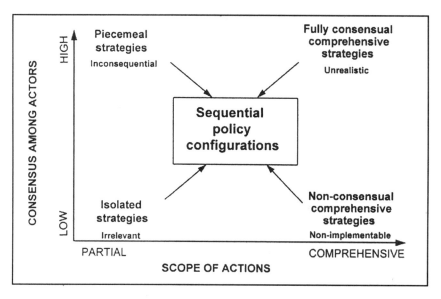

During the past few years, the American continent has witnessed experiences in the different reform strategies. In general, the four extreme alternatives shown in Figure 2.7 have important limitations. The reform proposal from the Clinton Administration is a good example of a strategy based on a comprehensive set of actions with an attempt to obtain a wide consensus among the major actors in the health system and in Congress. In fact, when all interested parties can openly express their positions, it is easier to obtain a negative consensus (on what they do not want) than a positive consensus. Therefore, fully consensual comprehensive strategies run the risk of being **unrealistic**.

In contrast, most past initiatives in the continent can be classified in the opposite extreme. Proposals have been focused on particular projects (a vertical programme, a hospital, a specialty or a region) without any real need for consensus. From the point of view of a systemic reform this strategy turns out to be **irrelevant**.

It has become increasingly frequent to find mixed strategies. One of them privileges the search for high consensus at the expense of comprehensive decisions. About a dozen countries in the continent have established national health councils as consensus-building mechanisms. Usually consensus is reached on broad principles (like universality and solidarity). It has proved to be much more difficult to achieve agreement on specific actions, since those affected by a decision usually have the capacity to block the actual adoption of all but partial changes. Hence, many of the proposals resulting from this strategy turn out to be **inconsequential**.

Finally, there can also be situations where authorities attempt to implement comprehensive proposals without achieving consensus. Typically, this has been a technocratic approach, often associated with the leadership of an agent who is external to the health sector. Several past dictatorships in Latin America have tried this strategy. Even though decisions may be made, the most common result is that the proposals remain as decrees, and hence they are **not implementable**.

As can be seen, all extreme strategies exhibit serious problems for making or enforcing decisions. They are, therefore, limited in their capacity to undertake systemic reforms. As in the case of the health system models reviewed earlier, more balanced approaches yield better results. Change processes require consensus on the major directions and principles of reform. Once such a consensus is reached, authorities should have greater degrees of freedom on the concrete implementation of the general guidelines. More than seeking full consensus from the beginning or executing simultaneously all the actions that a systemic reform requires, it would seem that the probabilities of success increase with strategies that identify sets of coherent interventions to attack the most critical bottlenecks in the system. In turn, the efficacy of this strategy depends on obtaining the double consensus of beneficiaries and decision-makers, so that the process of change can have the endogenous support of the major forces, which can then neutralise opponents, and so that initial decisions can induce further changes to deepen the scope of reform. Indeed, the most successful reform processes have identified sequential configurations of policy interventions with high levels of technical quality and internal coherence, which are implemented progressively.

Conclusions

The present conditions of health in Latin America and the trends that are already defining its future all point in a clear direction: the need for a comprehensive reform. In this effort, it will be important to preserve the elements of progress achieved during the past half century. At the same time, it will be necessary to identify and supersede the obstacles to further improvement.

Reform must be guided by a systemic approach that looks at populations and institutions. In this way, it will be better positioned to address the double challenge facing health systems in Latin America: to eliminate the backlog of accumulated problems and at the same time to deal with the emerging conditions.

Present arrangements have proved to be incapable of confronting that double challenge in a way that promotes equity, quality and efficiency. Therefore, we have proposed a new model of structured pluralism. This is a pragmatic, 'centrist' approach that avoids the pitfalls of extreme arrangements while trying to strike a fair balance among the legitimate interests of all actors. This model seeks a progressive horizontal integration of heterogeneous populations in a pluralistic system organised by functions. For each of these functions, the model proposes specific innovations. Modulation becomes the core public responsibility centred on the development of fair rules of the game. Financing becomes the central mission of a renewed social security that is better adapted to the new economic, social and political conditions of Latin America. Articulation becomes an opportunity for creative improvement based on instruments to mediate transactions. Delivery becomes a space for introducing pluralism with the right incentives.

Thus, our proposal moves away from the present vertical integration of functions in a single organisation and the ensuing conflicts of interest. But we do not automatically adopt the simple notion of separating financing and delivery that is so current in the reform debate. In structured pluralism the separation of functions goes beyond a simplistic prescription and includes various modalities. First, modulation is differentiated from financing and delivery, which avoids conflicts of interest from the traditional vertically integrated Ministry of Health. Second, there is a differentiation between the purchase and the production of services, which opens the possibility for introducing innovative organisations for health services articulation. Third, while the separation between financing and delivery is maintained at the level of the health system, specific OHSAs can develop diverse ways of combining insurance functions with direct involvement in the market for health services.

By carefully learning from experiences in other parts of the world, Latin American countries can effectively 'leapfrog' in the development of structured pluralism. It would be unproductive to simply copy models such as European public contracts or Canadian provider autonomy or American managed competition. These have all proved to be valid strategies for their respective circumstances. Our model of structured pluralism learns from these experiences by adopting their positive elements and correcting their shortcomings, but most of all by adapting them to the particular situation of Latin America. Clearly, every country will have to carry this learning and adaptation process even further into the specifics of its own circumstances.

In this search for specificity, several conclusions stand out as potential guidelines for advancing health system reform initiatives in Latin American countries:

1. Institutional strengthening is an essential condition to achieve an effective division of functions in the health system.

2. Without fundamental changes in the configuration and operation of institutions, decentralisation will simply multiply bureaucratic structures and inefficient practices. Decentralisation strategies must therefore be rethought in a pluralistic framework like the one proposed in this chapter.

3. In attempting to introduce instruments for efficient management, global incentive mechanisms seem to be more effective and easier to implement than instruments requiring detailed micromanagement.

4. The development of non-bureaucratic forms of modulation and the promotion of OHSAs emerge as two fundamental strategies for future work in health system reform.

5. In the end, reforms must lead to a new equilibrium among actors in the health system, which corrects the multiple forms in which consumer sovereignty has been limited.

These are times of exploration and renewal. New ways of thinking about and acting upon health systems are emerging through the open discussion of ideas and experiences. By confronting the risks of innovation, Latin American societies will also be able to invent a better future for themselves.

Acknowledgments

This chapter is based on a paper that was initially prepared for the Technical Department for Latin America and the Caribbean of the World Bank. A preliminary version was presented at the Special Meeting of Ministers of Health from Latin America and the Caribbean on Health Sector Reform, organised by the Pan American Health Organisation, the World Bank, the Inter-American Development Bank, the Economic Commission for Latin America and the Caribbean, the Organisation of American States, the United Nations Children's Fund, the United Nations Fund for Population Activities and the US Agency for International Development, Washington, DC, 29–30 September 1995.

We are grateful to Philip Musgrove for his detailed and accurate comments, which served as the basis for revising the first draft. We also received valuable comments from Alain Enthoven, Miguel Angel González-Block, Enrique Ruelas and Javier Bonilla, as well as from the participants in two seminars where this paper was discussed, organised by José-Luis Bobadilla at the Inter-American Development Bank and by Xavier Coll at the World Bank.

The responsibility for the content of this chapter lies exclusively with the authors and does not reflect the official position of their present or former institutions of employment.

CHAPTER 3

Health Reform:
Theory and Practice in El Salvador

Núria Homedes, Ana Carolina Paz-Narváez, Ernesto Selva-Sutter,
Olga Solas and Antonio Ugalde

Introduction

It is almost a truism to say that institutions are continuously transforming
themselves in response to internal and external political pressures, social,
and cultural influences and technological innovations. Reforms can be
viewed as changes purposely introduced to improve institutional organisation and outcome. Health systems have always experienced changes and
reforms. In the past the World Health Organisation (WHO) has given impetus and support to reforms such as the reorientation of national health
systems towards the objectives of health for all or the strengthening of ministries of health for the support of primary healthcare.[1] In Latin America
since the early years of this century, there have been innumerable health
reforms initiated by enlightened political leaders, revolutions and also by
ministers and civil servants who just wanted to do something different.

The above comments are necessary to avoid the impression that
health organisations have been static during the last several decades and
are suddenly being transformed. Future historians could easily arrive at
this conclusion when reading about the myriad of health reforms all
over the world during the 1990s. What is unique today is that suddenly
a large number of governments are talking about Health Reform (with
capital letters)[2] grounded on neoliberal principles, that in low and middle income countries Reform is funded by international agencies and
multilateral banks and that Reform is being implemented with the assistance of foreign 'experts' who, in turn, are heavily influenced by the
ideologies of the funding agencies.[3] Studies from various regions confirm that the characteristics of Reform in different parts of the world
coincide to a remarkable degree.[4]

Health Sector Reform is immersed in a broader context of governmental changes that have emerged as a result of changing economic
ideologies, donor pressures and fiscal constraints.[5] It is well known that

---

[1] Kutzin (1995).
[2] In this chapter the authors have used capital letters when referring to the neoliberal Health
Reform designed, marketed and financed by international agencies under the leadership of the
World Bank.
[3] Mills (1998a).
[4] Pan American Health Organisation (1997); Kutzin (1995).
[5] BID et al. (1996), pp. 10–13.

most Latin American countries suffered economic recessions of varying severity in the late 1970s and that they had serious difficulties in repaying their loans. As a condition for new lending to bail countries out, the World Bank and the International Monetary Fund (IMF) forced governments to carry out structural adjustments. In addition, these two institutions advocated a reduction in the size of state expenditures and induced governments to rethink their functions. It has been argued that under its new role the state should no longer provide services but rather regulate the provision of services by the private sector. Health Reform follows the same principles: to encourage private sector involvement, use public sector funds to purchase privately provided services; decentralisation of government; and reduction of public health financing.[6]

In this chapter we first identify the preconditions or enabling factors we consider to be necessary for the success of health reforms. A critical analysis of the theoretical principles upon which Health Reform is grounded follows. Finally, we examine the practice of Reform in El Salvador and from this analysis we add new insights to our assessment of the neoliberal Health Reform.

Health Reform Theory

Pre-conditions for Health Reform success

Not all reforms are successful; in fact history shows that success is more the exception than the rule. More and more scholars are attempting to identify the factors that facilitate or preclude the success of a given intervention. The outcome of earlier reforms in Latin America suggests that health reforms cannot be successful without previous substantial changes in the basic structure of the public sector. The political, social and economic characteristics of Latin American countries vary widely and we do not aim to discuss the feasibility of each country's Health Reform. The only purpose is to identify some basic factors that may be required for a successful implementation.

We argue that successful reforms need to respond to national/local initiatives, to be grounded on local values and that citizens need to be actors, not just objects of a reform. Other important aspects relate to how existing government structures support the implementation of Reform (if, for example, the political, judicial and law enforcement systems have the capacity to carry out the responsibilities attached to the reform) and if the country has the technical skills and the financial ability to implement the reform.

In Latin America the current Health Reform has been promoted by international agencies that have played a major role in its design; consequently, they tend not to be based on local values. The similarity of the reforms in all countries confirms this view. Privatisation of health services, understood as the transfer of the responsibility for the provision of health

---

[6] Pan American Health Organisation (PAHO, 1997); Bossert et al. (1998).

services from the public to the private sector, is one of the basic principles of the Health Reform but could contradict the right to health expressed in most Latin American Constitutions.[7] Health Reform has not been participatory. Researchers suggest that associations representing various interest groups (such as health professional associations, labour unions, political parties, peasant organisations and NGOs) have voiced their disappointment at the secrecy in which Reform has been conceived.[8] It is well known that in most Latin American countries law enforcement and judicial systems are very weak and in some countries they have almost collapsed. Scholars who have studied the technical and financial implementability of Reform have raised serious concerns regarding the financial sustainability and ability of governments to regulate the sector.

Theoretical principles: expected impact and immediate strategies

The objectives of Health Reform are broad and widely accepted: greater equity and efficiency, improved quality of care (hopefully leading to improved health status) and greater consumer satisfaction; all within a framework of financial soundness and long-term sustainability (Column 1 of Table 3.1). In fact there is not much new here: any health system design would specify the same objectives. What might be more controversial are the proposed strategies (Column 2 of Table 3.1),[9] which include any combination of the following: reorientation of functions of the public health sector; decentralisation of decision-making and greater community participation; downsizing of the government apparatus by privatising the provision of services; the introduction of basic packages of services; financial reforms (increasing the share of private financing); and managerial improvements. While there is no question that management needs to improve, the likelihood that the rest of the proposed strategies will assist in achieving the intended impact is questionable.

According to the Health Reform theory advanced by the multilateral organisations under the leadership of the World Bank, in reformed health systems ministries would no longer provide health services directly; instead their roles would be reduced to assess needs, define policies, establish and enforce regulations and ensure that the private sector delivers health services efficiently (Box 1, Col. 2). To carry out the new functions ministries of health would need to change their skill mix and personnel attitudes. However, the identification of the new skills, the design of the training programmes and the training of new administrators has by and large been overlooked (Box 6, Col. 3). The implementation of Health Reform confirms that greater reliance on market mechanisms requires more regulation, not less. The establishment of regulatory mechanisms requires appropriate legislation, procedures and the creation of regulatory agencies. It is doubtful

---

[7]   Editorial (1998); Pan American Health Organisation (1998).

[8]   Acosta et al. (1998); Bossert et al. (1998); Icú (1998); Verdugo (1998).

[9]   Based on how Reform progress is being measured, it appears that the proposed strategies are becoming the goals of the reform.

that in most Latin American countries ministries by themselves can satis-factorily perform these functions.

Table 3.1: Expected Health Reform Impact, Strategies (Goals), Over-looked Strategies and Process Impact

Expected impact	Immediate strategies/goals	Overlooked strategies	Observed Impact
Column 1	Column 2	Column 3	Column 4
1. Equity	1. Reorientation of functions of the public sector (regulatory/supervisory roles)	Health promotion and prevention, information, education and communication (IEC)	1. Creation of Reform units as parallel decision-making structures
2. Efficiency	2. Decentralisation/community participation	2. Environmental health	2. Termination of indigenous reforms
3. Quality	3. Downsizing/privatisation	3. Occupational health	3. Negative impact on public sector management: brain drain, demoralisation, etc.
4. Consumer satisfaction	4. Financial reforms	4. Control of advanced technology	4. Increased debt
	5. Basic health packages	5. Adequate use of drugs (essential drugs, basic lists)	
	6. Managerial improvements	6. Human resources training and management	

Decentralisation is one of the pillars of Health Reform (Box 2, Column 2). A growing body of literature suggests that decentralisation as implemented is not producing the intended results. Decentralisation tends to increase inequity, exacerbate regional and social class disparities and reduce the quality of care,[10] in part because the lower administrative levels do not have the resources and personnel to provide care at the same level that was offered before decentralisation, and because some communities are politically more powerful than others and can extract more resources from the state and central governments.[11] In addition, decentralisation will increase administrative costs if central level budgets are not reduced when decentralised administrative structures are created. Moreover, Health Reform strategists have assumed that decentralisation would promote community participation, but frequently community participation is controlled by local elites who defend their own interests at the expense of the other members of the community.[12]

Privatisation is another basic component of Health Reform that does not seem to be contributing to higher equity and efficiency, nor to better quality of care for the majority. Studies in Chile, Brazil, Nicaragua and Guatemala have shown that privatisation favours wealthy patients and that private insurance firms are reaping large benefits. Through a variety of mechanisms the public sector subsidises the private premiums of affluent citizens while the services offered to the poor have decreased significantly.[13] We would like to label this type of privatisation 'selective privatisation' because it benefits the wealthy at the expense of the poor.

Contrary to the theoretical postulates, privatisation does not always contribute to competition because in rural areas it is not possible to have competing providers, not even for primary care, and reasons of efficiency and geographical distance severely curtail the possibility of hospital competition in most urban centres. Lack of competition, the absence of an appropriate regulatory environment and corruption in the private sector explain why improvements in efficiency have not followed privatisation.[14] The private sector may not have the infrastructure to offer services to the health sector even for ancillary services. Community-based insurance schemes do not eliminate financial access problems and user fees tend to exclude the poor more than the rich from using health services.[15] Only under rare circumstances can user fees improve the quality of services, as when the fees are retained at the health facility and there is managerial capacity at the local level.

The concept of basic health packages (Box 5, Column 2) is similar to that of selective primary care, which has been severely criticised by health experts because it distorts the spirit of Alma Ata.[16] Because of alleged financial constraints, international agencies recommend that governments select a few in-

---

[10] Jané Camacho (1999); Gershberg (1998); Larrañaga (1997a); González-Block (1989); Conyers (1983).
[11] Engs et al. (1990).
[12] Ugalde (1998 and 1985); OPS (1984).
[13] Jané Camacho (1999); Wainer (1997).
[14] Rodrigues (1989).
[15] Kutzin (1995), pp. 9–20.
[16] MacDonald (1993); Chen (1988); Banerji (1984); and Briscoe (1984).

UNIVERSITY OF HERTFORDSHIRE LRC

terventions that could be offered to the entire population and free to the indigent.[17] The argument has been made that basic health packages are of
greater benefit to politicians than to the population. They allow politicians to
say that they are doing something for the poor while current patterns of inequity, waste, mismanagement and pilfering continue. If waste and mismanagement were reduced, most Latin American countries would be in a position
to offer a universal and comprehensive package of services.[18] There is no empirical evidence to illustrate that reducing services to a basic package may
have a positive impact on equity. The opposite might be the case: the percentage of health expenditures allocated to the poor may decrease.

There are other reasons for questioning whether the real intent of
Health Reform is to improve the health status of the population. Health
Reform is focusing almost exclusively on medical care to the detriment
of other strategies that are known to be more cost-effective at improving
the health conditions of the population (Boxes 1-2-3, Column 3). Ensuring that all citizens have access to quality medical care has little impact on the reduction of main health risk factors such as unsafe
environments, unhealthy personal behaviour and poverty. Even within
the medical care paradigm, the Reform model excludes strategies
proven to have resulted in substantial cost-savings, such as controls in
the purchase and use of high technology equipment and the use of essential lists of generic drugs (Boxes 4 and 5, Column 3). It ignores the
fact that physicians are inappropriately trained to resolve the health
problems most prevalent in the developing world (Box 6, Column 3)[19]
and that supply-induced demand, especially by the excessive number of
specialists in many developing countries, increases costs.[20]

In addition, Reform has created parallel decision-making structures
(Box 1, Column 4), is costly and could have negative consequences for
successful ongoing indigenous programmes (Box 2, Col. 4).[21] Reform
process creates uncertainty, confusion and demoralisation among civil
servants,[22] resulting in further deterioration of the sector (Box 3, Column 4). Furthermore, loans to pay for Health Reform increase the in-
debtedness of the public sector (Box 4, Column 4).

These general observations will now be examined in more detail with
reference to a recent Health Reform initiative in El Salvador. The case
study will look at the strategies used and the expected and observed im-
pacts and will identify overlooked alternatives. This will either confirm
or modify the critical assessment summarised in the preceding pages

---

[17] Warren (1988).
[18] Jané Camacho (1999); Ugalde and Homedes (1988); Ugalde, Homedes and Rochwerger
(1988); and McDonald (1994)
[19] Olubo (1994); Yesudian (1994); MacDonald (1993).
[20] World Bank (1987).
[21] Icú (1998); Verdugo (1998); Gershberg (1998).
[22] Bossert et al. (1998); Buse and Gwin (1998).

and will add new insights to those of other scholars who are examining the Health Reform in other parts of the world.

The context

Socioeconomic background

El Salvador is the smallest Central American country (20,742km^2) with a total population of approximately six million people (1998) and the highest population density in the Americas (258 inhabitants per square km). Rural dwellers represent about 43 per cent of the population and pressure on the land has been a persistent source of conflict and violence between the landless peasantry and the *latifundia* owners.

El Salvador had a GNP per capita of US$1610 in 1995. During the immediate years after the 1981–91 war, the economy expanded rapidly, with a real growth of seven per cent in 1992 and 1993 and six per cent in 1994 and 1995, but in 1996 it decelerated to three per cent.[23] In spite of this income growth, the purchasing power of low-income groups has not improved and food prices have risen faster than other goods and services. In El Salvador, as in the majority of Latin American countries, income distribution is characterised by a large concentration of resources in the hands of a small and powerful elite. The income of the poorest 40 per cent is about 16 per cent of the total income, while the income of the top decile is about 30 per cent.[24] Laure (1993) found that in the metropolitan area of El Salvador almost 50 per cent of all households were classified as living in poverty, of which 17 per cent lived in extreme poverty. There are no reliable data on unemployment and underemployment, but urban estimates place the level of open unemployment at around ten per cent and underemployment at about 49 per cent.[25]

Historical background of the civil war and political context

Two features have marked the recent political history of El Salvador: state violence and domination by the United States, which traditionally has exercised its regional hegemony through the local military.[26] Between 1931 and 1980 all presidents were members of the armed forces and the oligarchy was content to reap economic benefits and willing to forgo political power. The national budget reflected this militarisation; as an average the armed forces received more than 20 per cent of the budget. The military was not able to initiate meaningful social reforms; instead it increased sociopolitical polarisation and state violence. Thousands of leaders from political parties, labour unions, the Catholic Church, cooperatives and peasant organisations were killed and a culture of political violence and terror became part of the country's landscape.

---

[23] Pan American Health Organisation (1998).
[24] ANSAL (1994).
[25] Briones (1991); Ministerio de Planeación (1990).
[26] Blum (1986); McClintock (1985); Dunkerley (1982); Pearce (1982); and Gerassi (1963).

The level of political violence, which had intensified since 1972, became on 10 January 1981 a full blown civil war between the Frente Farabundo Martí para la Liberación Nacional (FMLN), alongside a coalition of leftist guerrilla movements, and the military backed by the USA. By the end of January 1981, the FMLN had carried out more than 600 military actions, including blocking roads, ambushes, sieges, attacks on military garrisons, battles and the occupation of towns and radio stations. By the end of February the FMLN had gained control of 121 towns and villages and had engaged in 156 battles.[27] The government of El Salvador let the USA know that, without massive assistance, the revolutionary forces would take over the country within a relatively short period of time and very soon it became clear to the contending parties that neither could obtain a quick victory in the battlefields.

The stalemate continued until the 1989 presidential election, which was won by ARENA, a rightist political party. Its leaders understood the futility and the high costs of continuing a war that could not be won by military means and so they opted for peace talks, which under UN mediation brought about a peace agreement in January 1992. The agreement set the foundations for the physical, economic and institutional reconstruction of the country.[28]

Post-war health conditions and organisation of health services

During the war, the contending parties declared immunisation truces that allowed the maintenance of relatively high levels of children's immunisation rates, and only one year after the war, more than 80 per cent of children were completely immunised against tuberculosis (TB), diptheria, polio and tetanus (DPT), polio and measles. The FMLN, with assistance from mostly European international volunteers, organised a health system based on primary care principles and health promoters that efficiently provided quality care to the population.[29] The World Food Programme and the US government supplied large amounts of food rations to the government that minimised the level of malnutrition brought about by the war.[30] A 1993 nutrition survey confirmed that extreme malnutrition of children three to 59 months of age was rare (0.3 per cent weight by height in 1993), and that only 8.7 per cent of infants with diarrhoea received no treatment.[31] The above explains why during the war some of the basic health indicators, such as life expectancy and infant mortality, continued to improve.[32] In 1998 life expectancy was estimated at 69.6, and according to the most reliable postwar source, in 1993 infant mortality was 41 per 1,000 live births.[33] An important programme ensuing from the peace agreement was the deactiva-

---

[27] For a description and analysis of the civil car, see Montgomery (1995); Editorial (1981); and Martín Baró (1981).
[28] Estudios Centroamericanos (1992).
[29] Lara et al. (1994).
[30] Garst and Barry (1990).
[31] FESAL–93 (1994).
[32] Pan American Health Organisation (1998).
[33] FESAL–93 (1994).

tion of the 10,000 antipersonnel mines left in the fields. In order to achieve this goal the armed forces and the FMLN provided maps with the location of the mined fields and by 1994 deactivation was completed.[34]

Nevertheless, the war had some lasting negative health consequences. In addition to the estimated 80,000 deaths, the war left several thousand disabled persons. There is no reliable information on the number and types of disabilities in El Salvador, but a census of war-related physical disabilities carried out as part of the peace agreement identified 12,114 war-disabled persons.[35]

Today so called 'external causes' (accidental injuries, homicides and suicides) are the main cause of death for adolescents (46 per cent for the age group ten to 14, 67 per cent for the age group 15 to 19) and adults (35 per cent for the age group 20 to 59),[36] and El Salvador has the highest rate of homicides in the Americas, about 120 per 100,000. Violence has become not only the main cause of death but also the most serious social problem in the country.[37] The prevailing culture of violence has many causes, but many factors can be traced directly or indirectly to the war.[38] Examples of direct causes include the countless cases of extreme brutality committed principally by the armed forces[39] and the large number of arms that remained after the end of the conflict in the hands of former combatants. An indirect example is the war-caused displacement of youths to the USA.[40] While in this country, some became gang members and on their return to El Salvador they engaged in criminal activities.

About 20 per cent of the population, almost one million people, were internally or externally displaced during the war, creating a variety of social and health problems.[41] A national health survey of mental health problems has not been carried out in El Salvador, but case studies suggest that the mental health problems caused by war atrocities and casualties and the displacement of populations are numerous and in many cases extremely severe.[42]

Not all the leading health problems in El Salvador result from the country's experience of conflict. As elsewhere in Latin America, El Salvador is experiencing an epidemiological transition characterised by increasing rates of chronic diseases (cancer, cardiovascular) and high rates of some communicable diseases, which in the case of some diseases such as Chagas', TB and malaria continue to rise. There are also recurrences of significant epidemic outbreaks of dengue and cholera.[43] The environmental degrada-

---

[34] UNICEF (1995).
[35] COPAZ (1993).
[36] Pan American Health Organisation (1998).
[37] Instituto Universitario de Opinión Pública (1998).
[38] Bran (1998).
[39] McClintock (1985).
[40] Cruz (1998); Portillo (1998).
[41] Morel (1991); Cagan and Cagan (1991); Lundgren and Lang (1989).
[42] Oakes (1998); PNUD (1994).
[43] Pan American Health Organisation (1998).

tion of the country has been considered extremely serious. Practically all surface water is contaminated by chemical products from agricultural fertil-isers, pesticides, herbicides and urban runoffs, and some studies suggest that soon the main aquifers will be chemically contaminated.[44] Officially, 78 per cent of the urban and 24 per cent of the rural populations are served with water,[45] but it is not known what percentage of the water is potable.

Theoretically, the healthcare of the majority of the population (about 80 per cent) falls under the responsibility of the Ministry of Health's (MoH) network of hospitals and clinics.[46] The real coverage is small due to patients' difficulties in paying cost recovery fees, geographical dis-tance and the poor quality of some services. The social security scheme provides health services to 17 per cent of the population, and a little more than two per cent are covered by other public insurance schemes such as those of the telephone and electric companies, the public school system and the MoH. Because of poor quality of care and long waits, an undefined number of social security beneficiaries use the private sector or self-medication, and because of geographical proximity, some benefi-ciaries prefer to use the facilities of the MoH.

The practice of Health Reform

The Health Reform process

In El Salvador, as in most Latin American countries, the need to mod-ernise the public sector and render it more efficient, equitable and ac-countable to citizens is long standing. The economic downturn of the 1980s and the structural adjustments imposed by the World Bank high-lighted the urgency for reform. The signing of the peace agreement in 1992 signalled the beginning of the reconstruction/reform of the coun-try and of the public sector.

Reform of El Salvador's health sector is an ongoing and complex process, and a final assessment will have to wait until the process is completed. Our information derives from interviews with key informants, documents from the World Bank and the Inter-American Development Bank and the few government documents available.[47] One document is the official five-year Na-tional Health Plan (Ministerio de Salud Pública y Asistencia Social, 1994) pre-pared by the MoH. This Plan is the MoH's formal and very general response to the government's decision to restructure the public health sector. Five shortcomings of the document are: 1) the absence of reference to the broader institutional changes affecting the public sector, suggesting that the MoH had limited planning capabilities and was unaware of the external environment and the need for enabling factors discussed above; 2) few references to other

---

[44] PRISMA (1995).

[45] Pan American Health Organisation (1998).

[46] ANSAL (1994).

[47] Fieldwork for this study was carried out with funding from the European Union contract No. TS3–CT94–0305 (DG 12 HSMU).

public institutions that perform health-related activities; 3) silence regarding the private sector and public health insurance schemes such as the that of Institute of Social Security; 4) a lack of references to non-medical care delivery dimensions of health, such as preventive measures, environmental interventions and health education and promotion; and 5) no mention of the health sequelae left by the war. These observations suggest that the five year National Health Plan was not a *national plan,* that it had been prepared with little, if any, input from national professionals outside of the MoH and that it had a dominant biomedical orientation.

After the peace agreement was signed and once the geopolitical importance of El Salvador had declined as a result of the collapse of the Soviet Union, the US government began to reduce its aid to El Salvador and welcomed the World Bank's interest in financing the reconstruction of the country. European donors were facing high domestic unemployment rates and were also interested in reducing their international assistance programmes, and the UN and its agencies were themselves under severe financial constraints. The World Bank conditioned lending to the government's acceptance of its neoliberal policies, and other multilateral and bilateral agencies supported them to different degrees. The Cristiani administration (1989–94) and the early years of the Calderón administration (1994–99) embraced the conditionalities almost without reservations.

The Health Reform Group (HRG)

Although the government's manifest desire was that the MoH would chair the reformed health sector (as opposed to any other health-related institution) a unit outside the ministry was created to lead the reform process. This unit was known as the Health Reform Group (HRG). The government could have opted to entrust this responsibility to the planning department of the MoH and have used the opportunity to strengthen its planning capabilities. The reason the Salvadoran government favoured the HRG was to be found in the World Bank's preferred form of operating in the Third World.

Reform groups have been created in other countries where the Health Reform is in the process of implementation under the technical support of, and loans from, the World Bank. The World Bank's preference for working with autonomous government units and agencies has a long tradition. Many national planning agencies were created in the Third World under the Bank's advice at the time it began lending to these countries in the 1950s. The World Bank has always preferred to work with autonomous agencies because they are exempt from cumbersome civil service legislation. As a result, they enjoy more flexibility and can bypass limitations and delays imposed by civil service rules and regulations in personnel recruitment, procurement and reimbursement for special expenses. Because civil service salary scales do not apply to these units, the salaries of the technical staff can be competitive with those of the private sector. This facilitates the recruiting of highly qualified professionals who are expected to work more diligently than civil servants. An additional advantage is that these units are not accountable to the legislative branch of government. Therefore, they operate with discretion and, if needed, with secrecy, and their decisions, which often have profound political and social consequences, are not part of a political debate. The World Bank, under the rationale that its decisions are technical, prefers to avoid political debates over its policies.

It can also be argued that the World Bank and the government of El Salvador believed that an entrenched civil service, whose employees represent a broad political spectrum, could not be trusted with a neoliberal reform that is supposed to downsize the civil service. It was unrealistic to expect that a bureaucracy could change its own institutional culture and behaviour and suddenly become an engine of change.

In El Salvador the HRG began operations in 1994 and it became the main intermediary on Health Reform matters between foreign aid agencies and the government of El Salvador. The HRG was responsible to the Intersectoral Commission, which was composed of the minister of health, the minister of planning and the director of the Social Security Institute. The HRG was presided over by an architect and had a neuro-paediatrician as executive director: both were individuals without training or previous experience in public health and they had been appointed by the president of El Salvador. These were political appointments, not chosen because of their public health expertise but because they could be politically trusted. In addition, the HRG included technical members, two from each of the three institutions, but as far as we were able to ascertain, they played a minimal role.

Secrecy surrounding the reform

The information obtained from the HRG was limited because the few existing documents were not made available. Public health workers (in and outside of the ministry), professional associations and international assistance agencies agreed that the HRG was working in secret. One of our interviewees, who occupied an important position at the MoH, indicated that the HRG was not sharing its activities and ideas with units and departments of the ministry. According to him, public health personnel did not understand the process of the reform because it had never been explained to them, but he believed this was perhaps the best way because the more they knew about it the more obstacles to its implementation they would create.[48]

We attended various conferences organised by professional associations to discuss the Health Reform. Both speakers and audiences alike made reference to the lack of information forthcoming from the HRG. According to one knowledgeable informant: 'All NGOs know that the reform is on its way, but there is no public information about it'.[49] The president of the Medical Association (*Colegio Médico*) who had previously worked at the ministry as head of the planning department added

---

[48] Interview October 1995.
[49] *Ibid.*

that the Association had expressed interest in participating in the definition of the Reform and had requested information about it for more than a year. He acknowledged that there had been some consultation between the HRG and the Association, but he had not been able obtain any documents about the Reform, and he added that his knowledge was based on 'rumours and guesswork which led nowhere'. This is the reason why the Medical Association as an organisation had not discussed the Reform.[50] The National Association of Nurses was also very concerned about the secrecy surrounding the reform and the possibility that its members could lose their jobs through privatisation and downsizing.

One member of an important NGO commented that there were no documents which could be used to discuss the ideas advanced by the HRG, and that the only information available to NGOs were the notes from a workshop to which a few NGOs had been invited. At the workshop the executive director of the HRG made a presentation outlining the basic characteristics of the reform process. At one meeting that we attended, after a NGO officer made a presentation of the Reform based on the notes he had taken from the workshop, members of the audience expressed their disappointment with the lack of information surrounding the Reform. The health promoters who were present at the meeting and worked with NGOs were concerned about their future status and potential unemployment. The health office of the US Agency for International Development (USAID) was also worried about the insularity of the HRG.

The HRG's secrecy was against the principles enumerated by the government's declared strategy for modernisation and the process for reforming the public sector. In fact, the principles of openness and participation also appeared in one of the first documents prepared by the HRG, which we were able to access by accident.[51] According to this document, a modern and efficient state is participatory and should establish mechanisms to allow for greater participation. Communities should be the protagonists in eliciting the solution to their problems and should be the main actors of their own development.[52] The document explains that high quality management is characterised by 'systems of coordination and decision-making that are agile and participatory'.[53]

In an interview with the executive director of the HRG, we inquired about the reasons for the secrecy with which the group was carrying out its activities and the lack of availability of documents. The director indicated that first the HRG itself had to determine what was needed and added that he was not in favour of popular consultations similar to the ones carried out by the education sector. We were also promised a document outlining the characteristics of the Health Reform that was close to being completed. The

---

[50] Interview with D.J.M. Ticas, September 1995.
[51] Grupo de Reforma del Sector Salud (1995).
[52] *Ibid.*, p. 6.
[53] *Ibid.*, p. 11.

document was never made available, either because it was never completed or because the director preferred not to share it with us.

Why did the HRG's behaviour contradict the principles expressed in its first document? It is possible that the document was written by consultants, and the HRG did not consider it necessary to adhere to its content. Perhaps the intention of the HRG was to prepare the Reform without consultations and then seek an endorsement from the various interest groups and citizens. In their minds, participation may have meant endorsement of the reform with the possibility of introducing minor changes. It is also possible that, given the lack of public health experience of the members of the HRG and the extreme complexity of the health sector, the HRG made little progress or encountered unexpected problems. In the latter case, the lack of information and documentation would only be a manifestation of these difficulties. Another possible explanation is the concern mentioned earlier by one of the interviewees: civil servants need to be kept in the dark about changes that may affect them in order to avoid a fifth column and early opposition to the changes. This view is supported by the following statements written in the first HRG document:

> ... the need for a gradual process of citizen participation starts with an internal awareness-raising of the Ministry of Public Health and other public health sector personnel, and continues with efforts aimed at generating, shaping and maintaining a positive public opinion of the health sector reform ... A specialist firm will design a campaign to this respect; all other health sector actors will be approached with the appropriate instruments and social communication instruments will be used.[54]

The above document, which we can assume was prepared by or with the assistance of a consultant paid with funds from a loan or grant from the World Bank, suggests that the HRG saw the need to prepare the blueprints of the Reform with secrecy and without consultation. After this task was accomplished, the HRG would market the Reform utilising modern technologies and mass media. According to this interpretation, the expectation of the HRG was that once the population had 'purchased' the Reform, interest groups would not be able to derail it. The World Bank's understanding of participation seems to be more closely related to the concept of social engineering or manipulation than to democratic principles.

The first task of the HRG was to produce summaries of three existing policy documents: the Plan for Modernising the Public Sector, the 1994–99 National Social and Economic Development Plan and the 1994–99 National Health Plan. The World Bank had a leading influence in their content, although the National Health Plan had also some input from USAID, PAHO and other UN agencies. Using these documents as a basis, the HRG presented in January 1995 a first formulation of the Reform.

---

[54] Grupo de Reforma del Sector Salud (1995), pp. 39–40.

The second objective was to outline the inefficiencies of the sector, an exercise that the Analysis of the El Salvador Health System (ANSAL) — a multimillion-dollar comprehensive health assessment financed by USAID — had already done in 1993.[55] The list of problems identified by HRG was practically the same as those found by ANSAL: high costs due to low productivity; inappropriate technology; poor management processes; accounting and budgeting deficiencies; heavy centralisation; excessive curative and hospital orientation of care; and lack of coordination and duplication among different public health institutions. Many of these constraints had been noted in previous evaluations of the health sector of El Salvador and were not very different from those found in other Latin American countries,[56] which have been documented in innumerable studies and reports. However, both ANSAL and the HRG failed to find out why problems that had been identified repeatedly in the past had remained unresolved. Such an attempt would have led them to discover the absence of enabling factors discussed in the first part of this chapter. At least ANSAL addressed problems individually and advanced solutions for each; instead the HRG ignored ANSAL's recommendations and followed the neoliberal Health Reform packet designed by armchair bureaucrats in Washington.[57]

The content of the Reform

From the inception of the reconstruction, the government accepted the interference of international agencies in the national decision-making process.[58] The strategies adopted by the HRG included decentralisation, a reduction of the role of the public sector through the privatisation, the official approval of recovery fees and the free provision of a minimum health package for indigent groups. These coincide remarkably well with those of the neoliberal Health Reform.

Privatisation and decentralisation of the public health sector

The privatisation of El Salvador's public enterprises began in 1991, as soon as it was understood that a peace agreement would be forthcoming.[59] The programme identified three categories of state enterprises: those to be sold immediately; those to be sold within one or two years, that is after some restructuring; and enterprises that required major restructuring or that, because of political risks, had to wait for a considerable amount of time before being privatised. The public hospitals and the National Water and Sewerage Board were included in the third category.

---

[55] ANSAL (1994).

[56] Carneiro (1991); World Bank (1991); Ruiz et al. (1978).

[57] Ramírez Martínez (1998).

[58] Silva (1995).

[59] Prior to this date NGOs, particularly in rural areas and in regions under the control of the guerrillas, were providing healthcare. Some authors have interpreted the provision of health services through NGOs as an expansion of the private sector and a reduction of public sector involvement.

Throughout the document in which the HRG outlines the characteristics of the reform, it insists on the importance of creating a new smaller but more powerful health ministry but does not explain how to do it or why it is appropriate.[60] The document is also unclear about the characteristics of the privatisation and whether hospitals would be transferred or sold to the private-for-profit or to the non-profit sector. The HRG specifically refers to a non-profit sector without specifying its funding sources. According to the HRG, ownership of hospitals by non-profit charitable foundations or groups would render employees accountable to the local level and force them to be more competitive and responsive to the demands of the population. The HRG contradicts itself when it later explains that because of the special characteristics of the health sector, monopolistic or oligopolistic practices leading to abuses and inefficiencies may be inevitable. In view of this, the HRG decided that the MoH would assume the functions of controller and overseer.

In spite of the above, by 1999 the MoH had not privatised healthcare delivery. It should be noted that an assessment of the private health sector of El Salvador conducted as part of the ANSAL study reported that the physical infrastructure of the private sector, including hospitals and laboratories, was very deficient and that by and large it did not have the resources to offer a satisfactory level of service.[61] Also, the percentage of the population who can afford hospital and specialised ambulatory care is so small that the possibility of a for-profit private health sector in El Salvador is not foreseeable in the near future. Obviously, the idea of privatising public hospitals advanced by the modernisation programme of the public sector did not respond to an in-depth evaluation of the health and economic conditions of the population.

In 1998 the Institute of Social Security began to contract a few physicians for the provision of primary ambulatory services through a version of Health Maintenance Organisations (HMO). Each of the two HMOs approved in 1998 was given one geographical area in San Salvador and asked to recruit a specific number of social security beneficiaries and was to receive a fixed amount of money. It is too early to evaluate the programme. However, the selected physicians had little financial and organisational expertise. It was not made clear how the Social Security Institute would supervise quality of care, but based on the US experience, it can be anticipated that if the Salvadoran HMOs face difficulties in making an acceptable profit, they may opt to reduce service levels.

The second pillar of the reorganisation of the public sector is decentralisation. Historically, El Salvador's public sector had been characterised by a concentration of decision making. According to the HRG, decentralisation would bring decision making and control of public services closer to the users, in order to offer services more in accordance with local needs and make providers more accountable to citizens; as a result of these changes, quality

---

[60] Grupo de Reforma del Sector Salud (1995).

[61] Iunes (1994), p. 54.

of care improvements would follow. Additionally, payment for services would be a component of the decentralisation programme and further empower users to demand quality of care.

The HRG (and ANSAL) were oblivious to recommendations made 20 years earlier by international agencies affirming just the opposite. A 1978 USAID health sector assessment indicated that hospital autonomy and decentralisation was an impediment to planning and prevented the regional health units from carrying out their responsibilities.[62]

Perhaps the impetus for decentralisation in El Salvador responded to the same reasons identified by researchers in other countries.[63] According to them, the decentralisation of health services reduced central government expenditures by transferring responsibilities without financial resources to lower administrative levels. This policy fits in well with the economic policies imposed by the World Bank to recipients of its loans.

Originally, the plan called for the decentralisation of one department, which was to be used as a pilot case. From the experience a more refined decentralisation programme would follow. However, towards the end of 1995, each department became a health region and the capital San Salvador was divided in four regions. The decentralisation, which was little more than limited deconcentration, was hastily implemented and the new regional directors and their staff received minimal training. An evaluation of the impact of this deconcentration has not been carried out, but informal conversations suggest that the number of civil servants has not been reduced and there is little evidence that efficiency, quality of care and community participation have improved.

Primary healthcare and basic health packages

The HRG also incorporated in its programme the concept of selective primary healthcare, which in El Salvador had been promoted and financed for many years by USAID and in theory is a basic component of the World Bank's Health Reform.[64] Typically, selective primary care includes birth control and prenatal care, oral rehydration salts, child and maternal immunisation, some primary pre-school childcare and some nutrition supplementation for children of indigent families. The HRG followed the above selection, but by 1999 the basic package had not been extended to the entire population and relatively extensive rural areas continued to be deprived of some basic programmes.

The contradictions of the Salvadoran Health Reform can be seen in the fact that at the same time the HRG was advocating selective primary care, the representatives of the World Bank and the Inter-American Development Bank only gave this strategy token emphasis. The banks were preparing a US$100 million loan, 80 per cent of which — against their own clearly established policies — was to be allocated for hospital reha-

---

[62] Ruiz et al. (1978), p. 206.
[63] Verdugo (1998); Gershberg (1998).
[64] World Bank (1993a).

bilitation. According to a reliable informant, World Bank representatives had indicated that primary care interventions did not have much impact on health indicators and that they were not interested in lending for primary care. One of the Inter-American Development Bank's representatives clarified that the international banks preferred lending for hospital rehabilitation because they had more experience in hospital loans than in lending for primary care.[65] The banks' priorities reinforced the excessive emphasis on hospital care, which had been identified by previous assessments, including the World Bank's and HRG's, as one of the problems of El Salvador's health system.

USAID had spent large amounts of funds on selective primary healthcare through NGOs. The Agency viewed NGOs as the preferred means of privatising primary care. It was concerned that once its foreign assistance was withdrawn the few interventions provided by the NGOs would cease to reach many rural areas because of the MoH's inadequacy and unwillingness to provide the organisational structure, personnel and funding to maintain the basic services. As such, in El Salvador international agencies had opposing health agendas.

The reform process stalled

In 1996 serious conflicts between the ministry and the international banks emerged regarding the conditions imposed by the banks on the loans. The five-year US$100 million dollar loan was to be disbursed in two phases (40 per cent in the first instalment). In order to qualify for funding during the second phase, hospitals needed to comply with a mandatory management package which consisted of: 1) a utilisation review, involving analysis of patient management within the hospital, of coordination of admissions and discharges, of referrals to ancillary and diagnostic services, of emergency services and of medical records; 2) an integrated management information system that was to be standardised for the project hospitals; 3) a reform in financial administration within the hospital; 4) user-fee policy changes and reform in implementing fee policies; and 5) the creation of a management board to improve hospital management and the introduction of management incentives.[66] The ARENA government, which was experiencing a sharp fall in popularity and was concerned about impending assembly and municipal elections, was not willing to accept these and other impositions. The HRG was dissolved and the status of the Reform was left in limbo. Eventually, the Inter-American Development Bank withdrew from the negotiations and the World Bank reduced the health sector loan to US$20 million for hospital rehabilitation.

Discussion

As indicated, the Health Reform in El Salvador is an ongoing process and follows closely the Health Reform model presented in the first part of this

---

[65] Interview Oct. 1995.
[66] World Bank (1995), p. 14.

chapter. The few changes, which have taken place in the country's health sector since 1995 confirm our critical evaluation of the Health Reform model. The reform in El Salvador was designed without taking into account the presence of the required conditions or enabling factors. We have shown that the model was imported, instead of being grounded in local historical experiences and culture such as the model of primary care developed by the FMLN during the war; that it was not consensual, that is to say, there were no consultations with legitimate actors such as labour unions, professional associations, NGOs or peasant organisations; that politically it represented the interests of the conservative forces and not of the majority of the population; that privatisation failed to design mechanisms of control and supervision; that it did not develop programmes to train personnel for new responsibilities, as was the case of the directors and technical staff of the new health regions; and that it was indifferent to the possibility that a relatively large number of rural dwellers could be left without healthcare. Reformers did not take into account that privatisation was problematic, because the private sector lacked infrastructure and technical and managerial skills.

The strategies followed coincided entirely with those of the Health Reform model and the objectives were the same. The design of the Reform did not include a methodology to measure the impact of the selected strategies on equity, efficiency, quality and satisfaction, even though these objectives were repeatedly mentioned to justify the Reform, and our findings suggest that, as occurred in other countries, the opposite effects could result. For example, increases in recovery fees have made it more difficult for the poor majority to access services. Lack of services is particularly severe in some of the poorest parts of the country, which had been served during the war by the FMLN. During the last few years, many well-trained and competent promoters have started to abandon the health sector and to look for employment elsewhere. In part, the promoters' decision has been caused by the ministry's delay in recruiting them, as required by the peace agreement under the claim (made by the minister himself) that the promoters who had worked for the FMLN were all communists, and in part by the employment uncertainty created by rumours of downsizing. Without the promoters, local NGOs — the only providers of health services in this area — are finding it difficult to continue their services.

This in-depth study of the Salvadoran Reform confirms the impression that reformers overlooked prevention and other well-documented cost-reducing interventions. For example, the provision of clean water was never discussed by reformers in spite of the fact that most of the rural population and a significant percentage of urban dwellers do not have access to potable water, and control of communicable diseases such as malaria, dengue, Chagas' and TB was left off the reform agenda. The health reformers overlooked the severe health sequelae from the war. Mental health problems were ignored to the extreme of closing down — in the name of efficiency and downsizing — the mental health division of the MoH. Care of the war-disabled and the socially destructive and costly health problems caused by violence were not taken into consideration.

During the last eight years the government of El Salvador with the help of international agencies and foreign experts tried to modernise and reform the public sector, including public health and medical services. As far as health services are concerned, it can be said that the possibilities of success of Health Reform are not very promising. If the failure of Health Reform is not to have negative consequences, it would not be very relevant to document it, but our research suggests that the failure has had some very costly and undesirable political and economic effects.

As indicated, the neoliberal Health Reform has been implemented by a small group of political leaders of a Conservative Party under the influence of international agencies whose ideology they share. Politically, El Salvador continues to be very polarised. The day the extreme right loses political power and once it is recognised that Reform has failed, the new political leaders will reverse the course of Reform. When this occurs, the country will find itself facing the fact that Reform wasted time and money and that the reformers — ill-advised by international agencies — missed the opportunity to reconstruct a modern healthcare system after the war along the principles approved at Alma Ata in 1978. It was a unique opportunity because capital for the reconstruction of the country was available, as well as knowledge of the health benefits and cost-savings of many interventions. The opportunity has been lost, and the political consequences were recently well summarised by an insightful observer: 'The government is unable to bring decent healthcare or education to the majority of the poor. The war is over. But El Salvador has essentially returned to the conditions that caused it.'[67] Health Reform in El Salvador has contributed to an increase in social tensions and a return to the violent past by failing to increase equity, by neglecting to satisfy public health needs and by failing to increase the quality of medical care.

Several of the negative economic effects of the Health Reform have been mentioned in previous sections of this chapter. The loss of skilled health promoters, the time spent by civil servants preparing information for the HRG, the demoralisation of personnel and the ensuing productivity reduction caused by the fear of losing their jobs, the administrative paralysis resulting from the uncertainty of new policies and, of course, the payment of the loans which have achieved so little, all have economic consequences. The question of who should be responsible for the losses caused by the failure of Health Reform needs to be raised. Most industries return the money or replace their products if they do not perform as advertised or are defective. Perhaps, the multilateral banks should share the financial responsibility for costs incurred in the implementation of Health Reform that their staff design and market in poor countries when the expected outcomes fail to materialise. When this occurs,

---

[67] Rosenberg (1999), p. 55.

the banks should be required to cancel the payment of the loans and return the interest paid. It is time that poor countries begin to impose conditions on international banks.

The worldwide Health Reform that has been launched by international bureaucrats in many Third World countries without taking into account the different political realities, historical contexts and the cultural specificity of each nation may have unintended and unforeseen consequences for each country. For the reasons given in this chapter, it is unlikely that Health Reform will succeed. It will be in everybody's interest if the international banks stop exporting Health Reform and, instead, let each nation design and implement changes according to their own cultural values and historical traditions, managerial and technical capabilities, appropriate legal and judicial systems, financial resources and political commitments.

CHAPTER 4

Decentralisation in Practice:
Tales from the North-East of Brazil

Sarah Atkinson

Dona Ana, the district secretary of health, reflected on the recent elections for local government in which the party both she and the current district prefect represented had failed to be re-elected:

> There's a strange thing, my God how I wish the Getúlio Vargas Foundation or one of these big foundations in Brazil would do some research on this, because something strange happened, because all the districts which are most advanced [in developing the local health systems] and which most value this participation have not got their parties re-elected. Districts A, B, C, D – D, there the prefect has already been state secretary of health, he's a guy with so much vision, he's been the president of the District Prefects Association, travelled a lot, even been to Cuba and made a model district there in D and didn't get his party re-elected. District E didn't manage it, in district F there's my friend there, she's very progressive, didn't get re-elected. So you see, the people aren't taking on board the message; the mass of the population haven't taken it on board; this process is very slow.[1]

Dona Ana recognises an intriguing paradox. On the one hand, we have a model of health reform that is almost universally agreed to be the most promising way to improve effectiveness, responsiveness, efficiency and equity in healthcare provision together with social development goals of empowerment and democratisation. On the other hand, we have a suggestion that in districts in north-east Brazil where the model has been put into practice local populations have failed to recognise the benefits this offers and have rejected those associated with it. This chapter will draw out some themes regarding the nature of organisational behaviour and local political cultures and their implications for realising the health reform programme in north-east Brazil.

Two political cultures: the rational organisation and *coronelismo*

The Brazilian health reform programme was formally launched in 1988 with Brazil's new constitution, which, in turn, was followed by laws specifically regarding healthcare provision. The great inequalities within Brazilian society are proverbial; the provision of healthcare reflected these in the marked stratification in availability and quality of care for different population groups. The health reform agenda similarly reflects an avowed intent to confront and address social, economic and political inequalities within the context of a restored liberal democracy after two decades of military dicta-

---

[1]   Translated transcript of interview with the author, Ceará state, November 1996.

torships. Brazil is unusual in that a new commitment to health is spelled out in no uncertain terms in the constitution which asserts that healthcare is the right of every person and the duty of the state.[2] The main pillars of the reform agenda are universal access to healthcare, decentralised management with increased participation of the population in decision-making and a greater emphasis on primary and preventative healthcare.

The agenda for universal access to healthcare addressed the stratified nature of public health provision in Brazil before the new constitution. A major reorganisation between government ministries resulted in all publicly provided healthcare coming under the Ministry of Health in one system (o Sistema Unico de Saúde or SUS) and are open to all members of the population, neither of which was the case before. Having thus brought the various government providers under one ministry, the next major organisational reform was the policy for decentralising much of the management of healthcare provision to the district level. In 1996, the Ministry of Health was operating three levels of decentralisation into which districts could opt and for which they had to demonstrate different levels of capacity to manage locally. This was changed to two levels in 1997. Once accepted into one of the levels, the district signed a contract directly with the Federal Union via the Ministry of Health. On the back of this contract, an allocation of financial resources was made for ambulatory care or for hospital admissions. These were calculated on a formulaic basis that included considerations of both population need and system capacity. The minimum requirement to achieve even the lowest stage of decentralisation was for the district to set up a distinct bank account for the local health system, to develop and present a municipal plan for health, to develop a plan for human resources and to set up a local health council. In reality, the plan for human resources was rarely demanded, so long as districts demonstrated some awareness of the local issues in this regard. The local health council had to have a membership comprising 50 per cent health professionals and with 50 per cent drawn from the local population. Normally, population representatives are drawn from a mixture of residents' associations and other active community-based organisations in the district. This council is to be a decision-making council, not just an advisory council, and should be consulted to approve health plans, the annual financial reports and other such administrative procedures. The inclusion of a local voice into local health planning together with greater local autonomy over health-related decision-making are strategies commonly found in many countries' health reforms[3] and fit well with the rhetoric in Brazil for wider political reform.

The international literature on health systems development reveals few doubts regarding the potential benefits of decentralised management of healthcare. Moreover, the exceptions mostly draw attention to likely pitfalls in implementation rather than challenging its appropriate-

---

[2] Brazilian Constitution (1988); de Carvalho and Santos (1992).
[3] World Bank (1993a).

ness in general.[4] However, academic writings about the implementation
of policy increasingly indicate the complexity, confusions and messiness
this entails.[5] From the practitioner side, producers of explicit policy
statements and directives for health reform programmes implicitly work
with a rational systems model, a top-down approach in which policy
process moves logically and in a straight line from problem identification
through policy formulation to implementation and evaluation.[6] Thus
although a nod is usually given to the politics and values of different
contexts, in effect policy is represented as a non-political technology by
which to achieve apparently non-controversial, rational goals of effectiveness, efficiency and equity in healthcare provision. A successful de-
politicisation of policy indicates a successful establishment of a
hegemonic discourse on how a health system should look, either nation-
ally or internationally. Thus, despite a repeated assertion about the importance of appropriate solutions for different contexts, it is striking
how most policies for health reform in low and middle income countries
feature the same kind of rhetoric around decentralisation, participation,
quality and partnerships. This package of strategies largely emanates
from, and is certainly supported by, the World Bank.[7] Recently there
has started to be a louder call for this implicit treatment of policy as a
technology and of implementation as a managerial concern to be prob-
lematised and challenged by researchers.[8]

The very essence of decentralisation is to increase the space for decision-
making at the local level for the local level, so that the health system will be
more responsive to local needs and thus more effective and efficient in the
provision of healthcare. The nature of the social environments within which
such spaces for local discretion are created is thus likely to be a critically important factor in the realisation of the policy vision.[9] In the north-east of
Brazil since the beginning of this century oligarchic power, based on ownership of large estates has built up the system known as *coronelismo*. *Coronelismo* is defined as a system of local control, in which a small group
exercise control over the political, economic and administrative domains.
Social organisation and political culture are characterised by clientelism, as-
sistance-dependency, paternalism, favouritism and personal-links. Within
this kind of political culture, public provision of social services becomes a favour rather than a responsibility and the popular perception of formal
public spaces is that they are not public at all.[10] The return to an elected civil
government has opened up a new space for democratic discourses around
the nature of the state, local government, citizenship and inclusion. There is

4 Collins (1995); Bossert (1995).
5 See, for example, the collection edited by Hill (1993).
6 Shore and Wright (1997).
7 World Bank (1993).
8 Shore and Wright (1997).
9 Lipsky (1980); Pressman and Wildavsky (1973); Atkinson (1995).
10 Faoro (1991); Leal (1975).

a constant flux in the creation of political parties and political coalitions. Urban social movements have become institutionalised actors in the political arena and many new forums have been created to provide spaces for the expression of citizens' demands. The promotion of popular participation as a policy has been appropriated by all political movements, whatever their leanings, and thus the concept may be assumed to have different meanings and intentions across the range of political actors. Despite all this rhetoric about a restructuring of political space, there is a view, especially amongst academics, that apparent challenges to the oligarchic relationships in the north-east are only superficial.[11]

This lack of impact in the north-east of Brazil can easily be attributed to political inertia by the state level governments. However in the state of Ceará a political group formed by business people came to power in 1986 with a campaign slogan of 'the fight for the end of *coronelismo*'. This group has held power at the state level for four successive elections. They have institutionalised greater autonomy for local district governments through decentralisation and supported the implementation of the health reform programme.[12] Given this formal political commitment from the state level to the health reform programme, Ceará presents a suitable context for exploring the interactions of a drive for a new political culture spearheaded by a rational health system with the old entrenched political culture of *coronelismo*.

The rational health system: 'structures, processes and results'

The state of Ceará has moved ahead fast with decentralised management of healthcare; by 1996 88 per cent of all districts (149/184) had decentralised management of healthcare. The experiences of three districts in 1996 are drawn on to illustrate emerging issues: a rural district typical of the dry, interior *sertão* region; a traditional urban-centred district of the interior hilly region; and a commercial, industrialised district that is part of the greater metropolitan region of the state capital. These districts present three very different social realities within which the new decentralised health system was to operate.

The urban centre was the most advanced in its adherence to the reform agenda. This district was at the second level of decentralisation and tried to follow the directives of the reforms closely. The health facilities in the district comprised a private hospital contracted to provide healthcare by the district and a public health centre in the urban centre, together with a series of smaller health posts serving the rural surrounds. The district had established three mobile 'family health teams', which regularly visited underserved areas. The health council was established according to the reform guidelines with half the composition representing residents associations and other organisations in the population and half representing the health

[11] Palmeira (1993); Medeiros (1997).
[12] Secretária de Saúde, Ceará (1992); Tendler (1997).

professionals, public and private. The council met regularly every month to discuss the operations of the local health system. Ratios of healthcare resources to population were good by state standards (number and size of services, number of beds, number of community programmes), as were indicators of health and healthcare coverage (infant mortality rate, immunisation, clinical and dental consultations per habitant).[13] The level of satisfaction of the population with the healthcare was good (59 of 100 women surveyed, Atkinson, unpublished data).[14] The district health secretariat appeared well organised although the use of funds was not that efficient as measured by expenditure as a percentage of planned spending.[15]

The metropolitan district presented a more complex situation. This was a large district secretariat of health, highly organised into different departments with a good information system, efficient in the use of funds and well resourced in terms of number, size and range of services provided. There were in addition several private providers contracted by the district health system to provide healthcare. Yet in terms of health and healthcare coverage, the district figures were poor and comparable with the rural district.[16] The local satisfaction with the services was the worst of the three case study districts (41 satisfied of survey of 100 women).[17] The district was neither hostile nor particularly engaged with the reform agenda, had only established the first stage of decentralisation and did not have a health council operating.

The rural district had the weakest local health system of the three. The health system comprised a small basic hospital together with a number of health posts around the rural areas and a large number of community health workers. At the time of the study, the hospital functioned well but the posts were inadequately supplied with either equipment, drugs or personnel; indeed one had been turned to better use as a school, despite the fact that the district still receives money for its running. The district had achieved the first stage of decentralisation and had established a health council according to the reform guidelines of representation. Indicators of health and healthcare provision were poor although as mentioned above comparable with the metropolitan district apart from immunisation coverage.[18] Population satisfaction was slightly better with 45 per cent satisfied,[19]

---

[13] Iplance (1997).

[14] A survey was made in 46 districts of Ceará, including the three study districts, with a sample in each of 100 women from poorer neighbourhoods. Respondents were asked to rate their satisfaction on a five-point likert scale for five aspects of the healthcare process. These aspects were defined as important to potential users from previous in-depth qualitative interviews. The scores for each of the five components were added together and a threshold of satisfaction defined from the distribution for the whole sample. The percentage cited here as satisfied represents the percentage of the sample in any district that scored above this threshold.

[15] Data from Secretária de Saúde, Ceará.

[16] Iplance (1997); Data from Secretária de Saúde, Ceará.

[17] Atkinson, unpublished data.

[18] Iplance (1997).

[19] Atkinson, unpublished data.

although satisfaction studies commonly find an unwillingness among poorer population groups to express dissatisfaction in surveys.[20]

These quick, thumbnail sketches of the three districts depict an interesting scenario. The rural district looks reasonably good on paper in terms of a ratio of health services for the population, the recorded ratio of consultations for the population and the move towards setting up participatory structures within the district. However, over the course of a year following this district it was noted that in reality some of the facilities were shut and others barely functioning, that there were few patients and the population was, in fact, greatly dissatisfied with the health system. This casts serious doubt on the official figures produced regarding the productivity of the system, since little of such activity was observed in reality. Thus, something was intervening between plan and practice as regards implementation at the rural level. At the same time the metropolitan district with a far more sophisticated range of health facilities had surprisingly poor indicators of productivity in relation to the population and population satisfaction. The gap here lies between observed input and positive results. Finally, the urban district seems to function well and produce good results and this is also the district that most conforms to the reform agenda. This combination raises a series of cause and effect questions as to whether good healthcare led to this district being encouraged to take on the reform agenda as a flagship, whether good healthcare reflects implementation of the reform agenda or whether both reflect some independent set of factors.

Political cultures within the health system: views of the health reforms

A first step in trying to identify how factors beyond the rational health system might be interacting with its workings is to explore the meanings that the health reforms have had for those working within it, namely the health professionals. It is a truism that within any system and within any attempt to bring about change there will be conflicting voices. However, these different voices are not often explicitly presented in analyses of health sector reforms.[21] Among health professionals in the three districts in north-east Brazil, at least five types of discourse regarding the health reforms could be identified and mapped; I have labelled these the Egalitarian, the Compassionate, the Professional, the Managerial and the Disempowered. Each of these tends to attach to a particular group of actors within the system and the relative balance of each within a district can influence implementation.

The egalitarian discourse is that of the health reform movement. The moral superiority of this discourse comes from the desire to see a more equal society, including the right to decent healthcare for all citizens regardless of their socioeconomic status. The aims of the health reforms are seen as not only promoting good quality healthcare for all who need it but also as promoting democracy in society through the greater involvement of

[20] Fitzpatrick and Hopkins (1983).
[21] Atkinson (1997).

local populations in healthcare management. This was the dominant discourse heard in both the state level secretariat of health and in the district secretariat of health for the urban district. There was, however, a powerful alternative discourse also heard in the urban district, labelled here the compassionate discourse. Here the moral superiority comes from the desire to provide healthcare to the indigent, to those most in need and to those who have no alternatives. The aims of the health reforms are not discussed so much, but the effects in terms of limiting the amount of healthcare in terms of numbers of consultations or hospital admissions that will be paid for in any month are criticised. This was the dominant discourse heard from managers of private health facilities contracted by the district systems to provide services. Many of these facilities are private-not-for-profit and are religious in origin (the *santa casa*). Such private, charitable facilities are important providers, particularly of hospital care in the medium-sized towns outside the state capital. Many of the conflicts at all levels in the system, district, state or national, arise from conflicts over allocations of funding and are expressed as a conflict between these two discourses.

Two further discourses echo much that is found in the international health services and health reform literature; thus they have been labelled the professional and the managerial, and have some overlap.

The professional discourse expresses health professionals' primary concern for the quality of the healthcare being provided in clinical and medical terms. The moral superiority here comes from an emphasis on professionalism, skills and conscientiousness in providing healthcare. Before the health reforms, a good quality of hospital care was provided by the Ministry of Social Welfare (MSW) to those workers who were formally employed and paid compulsory social insurance. These facilities have been taken over by the Ministry of Health to make a single system of health, the SUS. The discourse maintains that there has been a drop in the standard of the healthcare provided and in the training that those facilities used to provide to health professionals. Those persons expressing themselves in the professional discourse were those who had previously worked in the MSW managed hospitals, which were located in large towns and the metropolitan region. While the emphasis here is on the quality of care that individual patients may receive, the managerial discourse expresses a concern with providing good quality healthcare for a district and uses the language of effectiveness, efficacy and efficiency. The moral superiority of this discourse comes from its no-nonsense, goal-oriented line of argument that stresses the necessity of getting the best value for money to address urgent health problems. There is little room in this discourse for the social development aspects of the health reforms that the egalitarian discourse espouses, nor for the individual and paternalistic caring line of the compassionate discourse. Here the focus is on doing a job and doing it well, which in this case means providing a network of health services. These two discourses were heard most among the health professionals in the metropolitan district.

A fifth discourse emerged from the rural district. Here the local prefect had in effect taken the management of the health system out of the hands of the health professional and kept control of it himself. The health system was barely functioning beyond the small hospital; few senior health professionals worked regularly in the district (physicians, dentists or nurses) and those that did felt they had little control over much other than the community health workers. Thus, there was a discourse of disempowerment of the health professionals by the local government.

Mapping these discourses begins to indicate some of the differences going on beyond the basic structural set-up and organisational procedures of the different districts. It is significant that the three districts experience and express their relations to the health reforms in quite different ways:

District	Discourse
Metropolitan	professional and managerial
Urban	egalitarian and (conflicting) compassionate
Rural	disempowered

Political culture beyond the health system: views of leadership, involvement and accountability

Three further sets of viewpoints have a potentially important influence on the implementation and results of the health reform and can similarly be mapped across the three districts. However, in contrast to the previous section, these are viewpoints that emerge from the local political cultures within which district health systems are established and operate.

The most striking aspect of local political culture as it impacted upon healthcare is the type of management leadership that is valued. Closely linked to this is the degree to which the local population resolve their health problems through personal contact with local leaders. These can be seen as modern-day expressions of the old-style *coronelismo,* in which decision-making and access to resources lie within the power of a few. Patron-client relationships are the normal way for poor households to gain access to resources such as health services. A personalised style of leadership is valued since this provides opportunities for potential clients to establish a patron for themselves. The continued importance of the patron-client relationship helps explain Dona Ana's paradox with which this chapter opened. Those districts that have driven forward reform agenda, with emphasis on the health sector, have essentially tried to establish institutional structures and procedures that apply to all persons in the population as regards the delivery of healthcare. This model of an impersonal, homogeneous system, or rational system, is long on rhetoric as regards democratising the social fabric of Brazil, but contin-ues to be at variance with deep-rooted values about the way things are done in reality. Thus, the party of Dona Ana probably made a mistake in overly neglecting the personal courting of the populace, at the same time as trying to challenge this very approach. The prefect who was elected was valued because he knew everyone by name, remembered details about their families and called at their homes, while on the managerial side he dealt with human resources personally, knew who was working on which shift and sorted out the staff leave himself. Per-haps this is no great surprise; the importance of patron-client relation-ships has been documented time and time again and the tendency for the reform parties not to have been re-elected suggests that nothing much has changed.[22] The interest lies in the variation between districts in the way these relations are expressed.

The metropolitan district had a far more heterogeneous population, having only developed as a district over the last few decades through rapid urban migration. The networks of patronage were not so immedi-ately obvious and were less embedded in long histories of relationships between families. Nonetheless, clear use of patrons to access healthcare was very common. Residents sought an aspiring or actual political figure in particular for financial help in accessing private healthcare or for transport into the state capital for treatment. Those working in the health sector thus had a special range of resources to offer, and a num-ber of physicians were politically active. The physicians did not, how-ever, dominate the political scene.

By contrast, in the urban district the handful of physicians certainly did dominate the political arena. The current and future prefect were both medical men; and other candidates and previous prefects were also physicians. The health sector in this district thus served as an excellent focus for political affiliations providing candidates with both the re-sources for patronage and a sphere of activities that demonstrates a care for the population's needs. There was no other sphere of activity locally that could generate the same degree of respect. However, despite the obvious valuing of personalised leadership in this district, the resort to patrons to resolve health problems was not so blatant as in the other two. Those working in the health system, although with political inter-ests and goals, also had a genuine commitment to healthcare provision. The competition between a number of physicians working in this district with political aspirations may have provided the drive for a smooth-working health system; the tension between the public and private pro-viders, described above with regard to discourses, may also have made health system activities more transparent.

In the rural district, patronage in its worst form was operating. When asked how they resolved health problems, people most frequently reported

[22] Eisenstadt and Roniger (1984); Gay (1990); Weyland (1995).

that they would go to the house of a political figure to get medicines; very rarely did they report that they would go to one of the health posts. Political figures were sought to help to jump the queues at the small district hospital, to see the physician or with transport to the neighbouring districts, which had more sophisticated and well-functioning hospitals. The prefect did nothing for the district, was hardly ever seen there and did not pass on funds allocated to the various sectors such as health. This district has already been characterised above as having a disempowered discourse about health reforms and health provision.

Two other sets of factors seem associated with the relative empowerment or disempowerment that the districts manifest with regard to the clientelistic relations within the society. First, the very use of patron-client networks to resolve health problems reduces the need for the population to combine and exert collective pressure for improved healthcare provision. One strategy of the reforms that aims to undermine the old patron-client hierarchical structures of Brazilian society is the establishment of local health councils. Only in the urban district was the health council functioning in any way similar to that envisaged in the policy documentation. Here the composition was a balance between health professionals and members of the general population. Meetings were held regularly and topics regarding the running of the health system were discussed. The council in the rural district had been completely undermined by the lack of resources held by the health system managers. Thus, although there was a council with an official balance between health professionals and members of the general population which met regularly, it had little control over the health system and nothing much to discuss. In practice, the meetings were also attended by the community health workers and became little more than team meetings for organising their work for the following month. Often the official council members did not attend; the council secretary would go round to their houses to get them to sign the minutes for the sake of meeting procedural requirements. The metropolitan district health managers deemed the idea of a council to be a waste of everyone's' time and did not hold meetings. This attitude is in keeping with what has been termed above the managerial and professional discourses with regard to the health reforms.

Secondly, the commitment of staff to the successful provision of healthcare in any given district can vary enormously. With one exception, none of the senior health staff lived in the rural district. The exception was the district secretary of health who was part of an important local family but at that time only came to the district twice a week to work in the hospital as a physician. There were no private practices run by any of the health professionals and none had any evident political interests in the district, not even the secretary of health. By marked contrast, the urban district is largely run by physicians all of them residents. A number of the physicians also have private clinics or laboratories in the district. There is a clear investment, involvement and commitment to the district by this group of professionals. The district provides their home, their livelihoods and their professional and political careers. The metropolitan district falls somewhere between these two. Although many of the senior cadres of health professionals do not actually reside in the district, they have worked there continuously for many years and have a greater sense of involvement and commitment to the district. There are a number of private clinics from which political figures have come who again can be seen to have vested interests in the district.

The nature of this involvement in a district is clearly very ambiguous. Various writers have commented on the negative effects where physicians have dual interests from working in both a public and a private capacity with the same population.[23] Here it is suggested that although these negative effects are not denied, there is also a positive side in that vested interests may also provoke greater commitment within the public health system.

Running through all these facets of local political culture are the values people hold about what is acceptable, and what can be done where leaders cross the boundary of acceptability. Again, the three districts emerge very differently. The urban district appears to adhere most properly to rules and procedures. It seems likely that this is because of the active political environment around the health system that forces a certain transparency upon the system. The population is aware that when unhappy with care received there are other, oppositional, persons they can go to with complaints. In the metropolitan district, people generally felt there was little point making a formal complaint because nothing happened. This seemed to reflect not so much a sense of disempowerment of the people but rather a sense of apathy of the health system. Indeed, people in this district had plenty of complaints that they expressed informally at health centres.

As mentioned earlier, satisfaction studies commonly demonstrate that urban and better off populations have higher expectations of the services to be provided and are more likely to express dissatisfaction with health services. A community-based study of satisfaction with healthcare in 46 districts of the state of Ceará found a strong, statistically significant association of high expressed satisfaction in rural districts and low expressed satisfaction in the large urban and metropolitan districts.[24] However, the population in the rural district discussed here did have many complaints about the local government and the running of the health services but quite explicitly expressed their lack of power to complain. The combination of complex networks of kin relations, the constantly shifting political alliances and the carousel effect of local politics (i.e. the ones out of power today may be in power tomorrow) were frequently cited as reasons for not standing up and denouncing malpractice. The only recourse to voice that the population had was through the elections for local government. The existing prefect's party lost fairly badly in the

---

[23] For example in Brazil see McGreevey (1988); Vellozo and de Souza (1993).
[24] Atkinson, unpublished data (1999).

local elections but an insightful motorist employed by the local government illuminated the nature of acceptable local practice. He said that it would be foolish to think that the newly elected prefect would not also be taking a personal cut from the resources of his office, but two things made him a much more acceptable candidate. First, he would bring in extra resources from the state level as he was politically affiliated with the state government and secondly, he would be active as a prefect and there would be visible products from his local government. This theme of how local populations define acceptable practices and where they draw the boundaries seems to hold much promise for further developing our understanding of how local political cultures influence the practice of health reforms.

Health reforms 'the Brazilian way' 'for the English to see'

Other writers have remarked on the particularly large gap found in Brazilian organisations between how things are said to be and how they are done, although none within the international literature on health system reforms. Caldas and Wood (1997) pose a challenge to orthodox organisational development theory by studying the interactions of Brazilian political culture with the introduction of western business managerialism and highlight numerous features related to the historical and cultural roots of Brazilian society that impact upon how organisations function: personalism; ambiguity; power distance; plasticity and permeability (with regard to external influences); formalism and make believe. All of these themes are evident in this comparison of variation between three districts in the north-east of Brazil.

Personalism is well illustrated by a saying attributed to a notable twentieth-century politician, 'everything for our friends, nothing for our enemies and for those we don't know or care about, the law'.[25] What is stressed here is the dependency that all have on personal contacts for operating in society; those without family or friends to call upon will have to have recourse to the law. There is therefore a tendency to concern oneself with individual needs rather than those of the wider community, since if you have a decent network, there is no need to draw upon the general principles and the law. This stands in contrast to North America, where individualism may be as strong but draws its strength from potential recourse to the law. The concept of power distance picks up on Da Matta's analysis of the common Brazilian expression 'do you know who you're talking to?'[26] Again, the central function of the law, or of accepted organisational rules and procedures are undermined by a widespread resistance to being treated in an impersonal fashion. Thus the expression indicates an attempt to establish some right to be treated differently, to be exempt from the rules as well as an objection to being treated as if any person. The operation of personal networks and an authoritarian power distance in Brazilian society act to promote heteroge-

---

[25] In Caldas and Wood (1997), p. 521.
[26] Da Matta (1990).

neity and inequality compared with North American law following which tends towards homogenisation and equality.[27]

More ambivalent in its consequences is the operation of the '*jeitinho brasileiro*', the Brazilian way, an expression for finding a way around the rules. Da Matta (1991a) points out how fixing up a '*jeitinho*' for getting around the rules should be seen as much as an institutionalised process as the rules themselves. The implications of this are double-edged. On the one hand, the Brazilian way undermines procedures that are intended to treat everyone equally by allowing unfair favours or by making exceptions for some. On the other hand, in a society where the rules may well disadvantage those already disadvantaged, the possibility of bending these rules offers a way to cope, to survive and to express resistance to society's structures.[28] Caldas and Wood conclude that in any situation there is not only what can and what cannot be done, there is also the '*jeitinho*'.[29]

The fourth feature highlighted by Caldas and Wood (1997) describes a Brazilian fascination with the other, the foreign. The society is thus highly permeable to external cultural influences. However, these external ideas, concepts, products and so forth are not merely appropriated, but are re-interpreted in the context of local meanings and values. In terms of foreign models of organisation and management, the formal structures and procedures may be put into place, but how the organisation really functions may be quite different. This final feature in practice has given rise to the Brazilian expression 'for the English to see'.

Together therefore, these features portray a political-cultural landscape characterised, on the one hand, by a disregard for procedures, strategies for getting round them built on personal contacts and a kind of institutionalised recognition that a way round them is necessary, and on the other, by a superficial respect for these procedures that leads to strategies to pretend that the system functions according to the rules. The result for an outside researcher is an apparent adoption of an internationally recognisable programme for health reform, including organisational reform, in the language of a rational system. There is also an apparent implementation of the reform agenda according to its prescriptions. Subversions of system function, failures to meet system goals and possible solutions are then quite reasonably sought within the set-up of procedures and rules of healthcare provision at local, state and/or national levels. However, in a society where the political culture operates specifically to ignore organisational procedures and rules, the researcher needs to stay around a little longer and watch a little more closely.

These features can go a long way towards explaining the two gaps highlighted earlier in the chapter between policy and practice in the rural district, and between practice and results in the metropolitan district.

---

[27] Hess and da Matta (1995); Caldas and Wood (1997).
[28] Barbosa (1995).
[29] Caldos and Wood (1997), p. 522, taken from Da Matta (1991b).

For this author, the interest in a study that focuses more on what might be called the political anthropology of health reforms lies not simply in highlighting the operations of political culture within policy implementation, but in mapping the different manifestations in different settings. The three districts featured in this chapter have indicated the variation that exists in practice in the space for local decision-making, local participation and system accountability. Why this should be is to be found in mapping the constellation of features of the local political cultures with respect to the implementation of health reforms. Thus, a tentative mapping is offered for the three districts in north-east Brazil.

The rural district: seamless integration

Personal links are everything. The local government overtly flouts the legal rules of practice but no one will denounce anyone else because of the complex inter-linkages of family and patronage together with the carousel of political power. Auditors are somehow satisfied, despite the fact that visits to health centres find them semi-functioning or in one case totally closed down. The health professionals have little commitment to the district. The health secretariat has no power over the local system but colludes in the appearance of operating according to the guidelines in holding council meetings, getting the minutes signed as needed, submitting productivity returns and so forth. Here we can see personalism, power-distance and formalism, or the Brazilian way, operating quite blatantly. There is much of the culture of *coronelismo* in operation, despite the lack of a large cadre of major landowners. There is a noticeable lack of any sense from the local population that any of this might be within their control to alter. A discourse of disempowerment as regards affecting anything extends to the health staff also. The health system is seamlessly integrated into the workings of the wider political culture of the district; the health reform rhetoric and policy have made little impact.

The urban district: comfortable coexistence

The urban district health system works well both in terms of implementing the reforms and in terms of its results. Here local government is dominated by health professionals rather than by families with long-established ties to the land. The leading physicians all live in the district and have private practices there. The private hospital, contracted to provide services, is antagonistic to the public sector and not hesitant to criticise, adopting an alternative discourse style. These vested interests in the fortunes of the district coupled with competition between the various health professionals for political power provide an almost institutionalised watch-dog style of opposition, which in turn results in a certain transparency in the health system's operations. This operates despite an evident culture of personalism seen in the value given to a highly personalised style of leadership, which was expressed the most strongly here of all three districts, and despite the potential conflicts of interests between public and private concerns of public health professionals. It appears that, although the dominant political culture in Brazil has several problematic features, it still may in some respects facilitate the operations of the health system. In this sense, the new reforms of the health system co-exist comfortably, possibly even synergistically with the local political culture. Whether this is durable becomes an important question. Nothing much has changed with respect to values of personalised leadership and its associated dependencies. It may well be that the reforms will only appear to achieve social development as well as health service goals in circumstances already disposed towards this kind of discourse. Nonetheless, on an optimistic note, there is a pressure for transparency coming from the health professionals themselves, and the functioning of the health council shows signs of a growing local confidence in the possibility of asserting the rights of the population.

The metropolitan district: bureaucratic isolation

The metropolitan district has only become densely populated over the last few decades. In this sense there is no local history, no local landowners and no personal networks established over many generations. The district is based on commercial enterprise and also provides a population to work in city centre enterprises. Thus the population itself is relatively mobile. Here the health system works in a highly professionalised manner with a view to providing good quality healthcare in the health facilities as recorded in the health professionals' discourse. Most of the professionals had little direct personal investment in the district although some had worked there continuously for some years. There were very many examples of personalised networks in operation but these usually depended on a straight exchange of favours, rather than rooted within more paternalistic interactions. The population was far more critical of the services than elsewhere, including the rural area where almost nothing was functioning. The health council was deemed unnecessary by health managers; however meetings within the local health system for staff and centre coordination were valued. The gap noted in this district is not so much between expressed local policy and practice, but between practice and results. This may reflect a lack of input from the local population as regards problems in provision. This local health system, therefore, seemed to operate in a largely bureaucratic manner with local political culture having relatively little influence for good or for bad.

Conclusions

The health reform programme articulates a vision of society in which there will be greater equality and greater democracy. The reorganisation of the health system is couched in the language of a rational model. This suggests that the main task, although by no means a trivial one, is to find the optimal arrangement of structures and procedures, incentives and penalties to result in desired outcomes with respect to effectiveness, efficiency and equity of healthcare provision. An evident gap between policy and practice and practice and results, both in terms of healthcare and in terms of political support in elections, leads to questions about what local influences are affecting implementation at the district level. Brazil has been characterised as giving only the illusion of operating according to the rational systems model, while in reality operating according to a range of strategies based on personal networks, rule-bending conventions and exercise of privilege. This characterisation is documented here as alive and well within the decentralised local health systems of north-east Brazil. The bold rhetoric of the new constitution and the health reforms is perhaps too optimistic that the political culture of *coronelismo*, whether in its old form or in new guises, will be easily undermined. Nonetheless, there do seem to be some changes afoot under certain circumstances that give some basis for a very cautious optimism, even if rational systems approach for health reforms and social change is misguided. A new mode of practice is needed that acknowledges the realities of the interface between political culture and organisational function, and which can find a way of both working within it and working to change it. Although a tall order, without this the reforms will function as little more than a focus for different allegiances through discourses, achieve little other than promote ever more illusion and reformers such as Dona Ana will continue to work for social change in vain.

CHAPTER 5

Getting Better after Neoliberalism: Shifts and Challenges of Health Policy in Chile

Armando Barrientos

Introduction

Health policy in Chile has mirrored the main changes in economic policy in recent times. The period after the Second World War witnessed both the expansion and centralisation of public healthcare into a universal, national service. The implementation of neoliberal policies in the 1970s and '80s refocused health policy towards extending the scope for private insurance and provision in healthcare. The return to democracy in 1990 has produced a reappraisal of health policy, with a subsequent emphasis on strengthening and improving public healthcare. This chapter examines these changes in health policy, the resulting structures of health insurance and provision and the unresolved problems and challenges affecting healthcare in Chile.

In the 1980s, health policy in Chile focused on extending private sector involvement in health. Private health insurance funds, the Institutos de Salud Previsional (ISAPREs), began operating in 1981 offering individually negotiated healthcare plans. The proportion of the population covered by the ISA-PREs increased to just over a quarter by 1997. They have attracted mainly higher income and low health risk groups and have concentrated on providing high frequency outpatient care. The migration of high-income groups from the public health insurance scheme, and cuts in government transfers in the 1980s, reduced the financing of public healthcare with an inevitable deterioration in service provision. Health policy in the 1980s resulted in large and growing inequalities in access to, and provision of, healthcare.

The return to democracy in 1990 was accompanied by a major change in health policy. The new centre-left coalition was committed to reducing the large inequalities in healthcare and to restoring the capacity of the public healthcare sector to meet the health needs of the majority of the population. In addition to securing significant increases in fiscal transfers to the public healthcare sector, the government has sought to decentralise healthcare provision and to restructure the internal mechanisms for resource allocation.

These major health policy changes of the early 1980s and early 1990s have provided both problems and solutions. Of particular concern is the articulation of private and public health insurance and provision. While the private healthcare sector absorbs a large measure of resources, the public healthcare sector remains the 'provider of last resort' as far as healthcare is concerned. This articulation generates many problems, which detract from an effective use of resources. Another concern, shared with many other countries at a similar stage of development, is the absence of strong cost containment incentives within the healthcare sectors. Finally, overcoming inequalities in access to healthcare continues to be a challenge for health policy in Chile.

These are the issues that will be covered in this chapter. The next section discusses the early 1980s health reforms and their background. The section that follows studies the development of private health insurance in the 1980s. The next section discusses the modernisation of the public healthcare sector in the 1990s. The main problems and challenges of health policy in Chile are then considered and conclusions are set out in a final section.

Healthcare reform in the 1980s

Healthcare reform in Chile was implemented as part of the early 1980s modernisation of the country's social welfare programmes.[1] The 1980 Reform of Social Insurance split off pension insurance and health insurance from other programmes. Pension reform introduced the new individual capitalisation pension plans to be offered by private pension fund managers, the Administradoras de Fondos de Pensiones (AFPs).[2] Health reform aimed to facilitate and encourage private health insurance funds in the shape of the ISAPREs. Within the public sector, the main thrust of health reform was aimed at decentralising healthcare provision and putting in place appropriate mechanisms for resource allocation. Compared to pension reform, health reform was more tentative and required considerable fine-tuning over the next few years, before it was consolidated in a new legal framework for the healthcare sector in 1986. The next three sections cover the background to the reforms, the reforms themselves and the adjustments made subsequently.

Background

Public healthcare developed in Chile as part of the services offered by social insurance funds (*cajas de previsión*). The earlier social insurance funds date from the 1920s in Chile and initially covered old age and disability pensions. These funds were set up for distinct groups of workers around a social insurance principle. Entitlement to benefits depended on contribution status and contributions financed benefits for specific contingencies. In the 1940s and '50s, the range of contingencies covered expanded to include first preventive medicine and later curative medicine. In 1942 the Servicio Médico Nacional de Empleados (SERMENA) was created to cover preventive medical care for white-collar workers and in 1968 curative medical care was added. Blue-collar workers were covered by the Servicio Nacional de Salud (SNS) created in 1952.[3] Over the next few decades these expanded to cover virtually the whole population, supported by increasing direction and funding from the government.

---

[1] Ministerio de Salud (1998a); Miranda (1989); Miranda et al. (1995); Superintendencia de la Seguridad Social (1998).

[2] Barrientos (1998).

[3] CIEDESS (1994).

An important feature of health policy in Chile was its stratification along blue/white-collar lines. There were differences across the two segments. Blue-collar workers received healthcare direct from the SNS providers, while white-collar workers had the option of receiving healthcare directly from SERMENA institutions or from approved private providers. If they opted for private providers, white-collar workers could purchase a voucher at a fraction of its value from SERMENA,[4] which was then redeemed by the provider. This feature of SERMENA encouraged the growth of private healthcare providers in the 1960s and '70s. Significant differentials in access and service quality across the segments persisted.

Health reform

The large-scale reform of health provision and financing implemented in Chile in the early 1980s belonged within a broad programme of structural reform of the Chilean economy and social programmes seeking to restructure these in line with neoliberal policies.[5] Health reform had as its main objective the expansion of the role of the private sector in the provision and financing of healthcare and the decentralisation of the public healthcare sector.

The first reform of healthcare, implemented in 1979, extended the option to use private healthcare providers to blue-collar workers.[6] It also restructured the SNS, attempting to separate its three main functions — health policy, provision and insurance — more clearly.[7] The Health Ministry (Ministerio de Salud) retained responsibility for general health policy and for the supervision and management of public health provision. Primary healthcare provision was transferred to the local authorities, the municipalities. Secondary and tertiary healthcare provision was also decentralised into 27 regional groups; the Servicios de Salud and the healthcare institutions within them were transformed into self-managed independent units. Public health services became the responsibility of the new Sistema Nacional de Servicios de Salud (SNSS). The health insurance and financing function was entrusted to the Fondo Nacional de Salud (FONASA), responsible for collecting mandatory health insurance contributions, together with government funding, and allocating these to healthcare providers as well as managing a voucher scheme for use with private providers.

This reorganisation of health provision and financing prepared the ground for the introduction of private health insurance providers, the ISA-PREs, which began operating in 1981.[8] Their introduction extended choice of public or private providers to the area of health insurance, as workers could opt to make their mandatory health insurance contributions to pri-

---

[4] Miranda (1994) reports that SERMENA copayment amounted to, on average, 50% of the tariff.

[5] Larrañaga (1997b); Marcel and Arenas (1992); Miranda (1994); Miranda et al. (1995).

[6] DL 2575 of May 1979.

[7] DL 2763 of August 1979.

[8] DFL 3 of 1981.

vate providers. The ISAPREs were encouraged to provide healthcare directly from their own institutions, or to negotiate service contracts with private healthcare providers. The establishment of the ISAPREs created two parallel sectors for financing and providing healthcare.

Fine tuning the reform

Between 1980 and 1986 a number of important changes took place aimed at facilitating the establishment and expansion of the ISAPREs. These included raising the mandatory health contribution level from four per cent of earnings to five per cent and then six per cent in 1983. In 1985 the Fondo Unico de Prestaciones Familiares relieved the ISAPREs from responsibility for payment of maternity benefits. Legislation implemented at the beginning of 1986 consolidated the new framework for the financing and provision of healthcare.[9] It eliminated the differences in healthcare for white- and blue-collar workers, by setting up a uniform compulsory health insurance contribution of seven per cent of earnings. This could be paid into the public health insurance fund, FONASA, or into one of the ISAPREs. Healthcare for non-contributing employees and for inactives remains the responsibility of the public health sector.[10] Copayments, already in place for FONASA beneficiaries who used private providers, were extended to cover the use of public sector health institutions as well.

Expanding the scope for private provision in healthcare

In this section, the impact of the 1980s health reform is examined more closely.

ISAPREs

The key aim of health reform was to extend the scope for private involvement in health insurance and provision. The ISAPREs, corporations whose main purpose was to provide health insurance and healthcare services, spearheaded this. There are two types: closed ISAPREs restrict affiliation to specific groups of workers, while open ISAPREs are open to all contributors. Large firms usually run closed ISAPREs, with services and insurance cover determined through collective bargaining. There are few restrictions applying to health plans. They must cover at least sickness benefits, maternity and child healthcare and preventive medical check-ups. Health plan contracts must cover a minimum period of 12 months and cannot be rescinded by the ISAPREs. Outside these requirements, health plan contracts are freely negotiated between the ISAPREs and the individual affiliate.

The ISAPREs have grown considerably since their introduction, both in terms of beneficiaries and resources.[11] Figure 5.1 below shows the population covered by the ISAPREs and FONASA.[12] The share of the population cov-

---

[9] Ley 18496 of November 1985, implemented in January 1986.

[10] Miranda (1989).

[11] Independent workers and pensioners can also opt to join a health plan from the ISAPREs.

[12] The other category includes those affiliated to the health fund of the armed forces, and to other minor private health insurance. schemes

ered by ISAPREs increased to 4.5 per cent by 1985, had trebled to 16 per cent by 1990, rose to 26 per cent by 1995 and has since stagnated.

Figure 5.1: Health Insurance Fund Coverage 1981–96

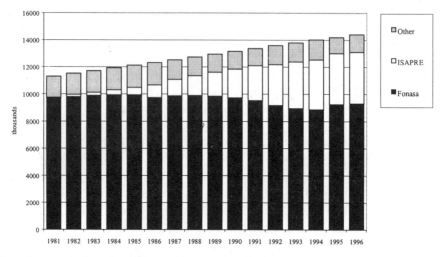

Data Sources: Miranda (1994); Ministerio de Salud (1998a)

The success of the ISAPREs depended to a large extent on successive policy and regulatory changes implemented by the government, which had the effect of encouraging the migration of medium and higher earnings workers to the ISAPRES. Miranda (1989) lists a number of measures that contributed to the enlargement of the potential market of ISAPREs. At the start of the ISAPREs in 1981, the mandatory health contribution rate was four per cent. This was raised several times to reach seven per cent in 1986, the current level. The government took over the payment of maternity leave from the ISAPREs, as this had been responsible for higher premiums for women of fertile age. These, together with a two per cent extra subsidy for low earning workers enlarged the potential market for ISAPREs.[13] At the same time, the copayment of FONASA beneficiaries opting for private healthcare increased, heightening the attractiveness of the ISAPREs for higher income workers.

The resources available to the ISAPREs have grown very fast, as they concentrate affiliation by higher earning workers. This can be shown by the trend in the ratio of the value of mandatory health contributions

---

[13] The extra 2% subsidy is paid by employers and discounted from their tax liabilities. This extra subsidy has recently been abolished amid opposition from ISAPREs as it provides them with around 7% of their contribution income.

paid into the ISAPREs relative to those paid into FONASA. It was 0.10 in 1982, rose to 1.1 in 1988 and thereafter to 1.94 in 1997.[14]

Key indicators for the ISAPREs sector in Table 5.1 below provide a picture of the sector. The number of ISAPREs in the market has risen, especially the open ISAPREs, but their number stabilises and declines after 1993. It is a highly concentrated market with the largest three IS-APREs accounting for 58 per cent of all beneficiaries and the largest five accounting for 76 per cent of them in 1997. There are indications that, after the entry of new ISAPREs in the early 1990s, the market is now becoming more concentrated. What is also remarkable is that the largest five ISAPREs have dominated the market since its inception.

Table 5.1: Key Indicators of the ISAPRE Sector

	1982	1985	1989	1993	1997
Number of ISAPREs	10	17	32	36	29
- open	7	10	19	22	18
- closed	3	7	13	14	11
Market share of largest three	81	48	50	50	58
Market share of largest five	94	69	69	72	76
Profits/operational income		4.8	8.3	4.7	3.1
Administrative and sales costs/operational income		25.6	20	20.1	18.9
Operational costs/operational income		71.1	74.7	76.9	80.5
Number of interventions per beneficiary		9.59	9.27	10.14	10.56

Data sources: Ministerio de Salud (1998a); Miranda (1989); Miranda et al. (1995); Superintendencia de la Seguridad Social (1998).

The financial situation of the ISAPREs as a whole shows that profits are relatively low (certainly in comparison with pension fund managers and banks in Chile), but the reported average hides considerable variation from the more successful ISAPREs to the less successful ones. In terms of performance, the administrative and sales costs of the ISAPREs have declined from the mid-1980s, but their current level (at around one-fifth of health insurance contributions) reflects the high costs associated with individual contracts and the need to shore up market share. In terms of services provided, the number of interventions per beneficiary have

---

[14] Miranda et al. (1995).

changed little over time: from 9.59 in 1985 to 10.66 in 1997. It is difficult to get a measure of costs per intervention, as the figures do not include beneficiaries' copayment or pharmacy costs. Commentators
believe that costs per intervention have increased over time for the ISA-
PREs, raising concerns over their ability to contain healthcare costs.[15]

Restructuring the public health sector

The restructuring of the public healthcare sector, involving changes to
both insurance and provision, was also expected to contribute to expanding the scope for private sector involvement in healthcare. The
health reforms extended the option of private healthcare and introduced copayment for the use of public sector facilities. The 1986 reform
established four categories of FONASA beneficiaries (see Table 5.2).

Table 5.2: FONASA Beneficiary Groups

FONASA Groups	Beneficiaries included	% of all FONASA beneficiaries (1990)
A	Paupers, pensioners, and those receiving family benefits	38.8
B	Low paid workers	30.6
C	Middle income workers	9.0
D	Highly paid workers	9.2

Group size data from CASEN 1990 (Mideplan, 1991); percentages do not add up to
100 as 12.3 percent of respondents did not know which group they belonged to.

Groups A and B can only access healthcare from public sector health institutions. Groups C and D can, in addition, access private healthcare
providers registered with FONASA. For groups C and D copayments for
the use of public sector institutions are ten and 20 per cent respectively.[16] Copayments for the use of private healthcare providers range
from 50 to 75 per cent.[17] As noted above, the increase in average copayments for FONASA beneficiaries raised the attractiveness of migrating to
an ISAPRE. Given that the mandatory health contribution rate is earnings related, medium to high earnings workers are likely to get a lower
copayment health plan with a private health insurer.

---

[15] Economist Intelligence Unit (1998); Kifmann (1998).
[16] Some services have different copayment. Primary healthcare has zero copayment, dental treatment
copayments are 40%, 60% and 90% for Groups B, C and D respectively (Mideplan, 1990).
[17] Mideplan (1990).

The health reform included the transfer of primary healthcare providers to the municipalities, with the objective of decentralising healthcare provision, providing greater autonomy and participation of the local community in the design and implementation of healthcare. In the first two years of the new policy over 550 clinics were transferred, mainly in rural areas. The acute economic crisis of 1982 ensured the suspension of transfers until 1987, in which year 880 clinics were transferred, with a further 419 being transferred in 1988. The municipalisation of primary care was strongly resisted by the health worker unions because it fragmented the healthcare system and led to marked differences in contracts and pay. A natural consequence of this change was the rise in inequality in access and provision in line with wealth differentials across communities, since wealthier municipalities made larger subsidies to their primary healthcare units.

The reform also aimed to introduce stronger incentives for micro-efficiency by supplementing historic cost budget allocations to health institutions with a system of payment for service. This was known as Facturación por Atención Prestada (FAP). It was supposed to reward institutions that increased their levels of services, and created incentives for local managers to raise efficiency. Its main limitation was that it only applied to a fraction of hospital budgets, on average around 20 per cent of their operational costs.[18]

Evaluation of health policy in the 1980s

The overriding aim of health policy of the 1980s was to extend the scope for private sector involvement in health insurance and healthcare provision. The restructuring of the public healthcare sector also brought in important changes, but these played second fiddle to the establishment and development of the ISAPREs. Furthermore, the impact on the funding levels of public healthcare of the migration of the higher earning workers to the ISAPREs, and a fall in government health funding, meant a deterioration in public healthcare provision.[19]

The focus of criticism of health policy in the 1980s was concentrated on the large inequalities in access and provision, generated by the reforms. The private health insurance funds attracted those groups with better health risk and earnings. At the same time, the groups with worse health economic risk concentrated in the public health insurance fund. It is not surprising therefore that the ISAPREs could improve on the services offered by FONASA for the categories of workers they attracted. A strong segmentation of the population by health and economic risk emerged directly as a consequence of the health reforms. Figure 5.2

---

[18] Miranda (1994).
[19] CIEDESS (1994) reports that public sector health expenditure per beneficiary showed a declining trend from 1982 until 1986. The slow recovery that followed meant that public health expenditure per capita did not recover its pre-1982 crisis level until 1991.

shows health insurance fund affiliation by income quintile for 1990, where this segmentation by economic status is evident.[20]

Figure 5.2: Health Insurance Fund Beneficiaries by Income Quintile in 1990

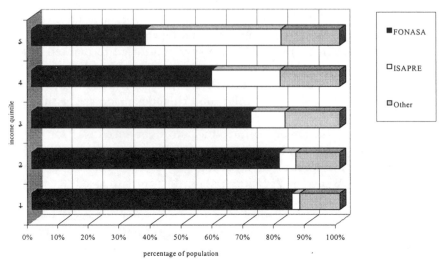

Data Source: Mideplan (1991)

The segmentation by health risk can be observed in the age distribution of the population across the different health insurance funds. In 1990, the ratio of ISAPRE beneficiaries to FONASA beneficiaries was 0.22 for the whole population, rising to 0.25 for the 15 to 59 age group, and falling to 0.07 for the 60 plus age group. The strong correlation existing between age health risk and economic risk reinforces this segmentation. In Table 5.3 below, the fractions of different age groups in selected quintiles of household income are examined separately for the ISAPRE and FONASA beneficiaries, using 1990 survey data.[21] As is apparent, FONASA insures a high proportion of older and younger groups in the lower income quintiles.

In part this segmentation is a consequence of the fact that the public healthcare sector is 'provider of last resort' and is responsible for delivering on the legal commitment to adequate and equitable healthcare for all. This justifies the large contribution made by the government to the funding of healthcare provision. In 1996, for example, fiscal transfers accounted for just under one half of public health sector revenues.[22] The ISAPREs do not share this responsibility, but to an important extent rely on this role being per-

---

[20] It can be argued that the reform eliminated the segmentation by occupational status only to replace it with one based on health risk and economic status.

[21] Mideplan (1991).

[22] Larrañaga (1997b).

formed by the public healthcare sector. The lack of adequate registration in the public sector enabled large cross-subsidies to the private sector, as ISAPRE beneficiaries sought treatment in public healthcare units.[23] These administrative failings encouraged and facilitated evasion and avoidance of health contributions from non-ISAPRE beneficiaries as well.

Table 5.3: Age-Income Profiles of ISAPRE and FONASA Beneficiaries in 1990*

Age Groups	0-5	6-14	15-59	60 +	all
ISAPRE beneficiaries:					
1st to 3rd quintile	0.35	0.33	0.24	0.35	0.27
5th to 3rd quintile	3.21	2.38	3.30	8.12	3.20
5th to 1st quintile	9.08	7.31	13.47	23.24	11.78
FONASA beneficiaries:					
1st to 3rd quintile	2.44	2.61	1.18	0.56	1.42
5th to 3rd quintile	0.25	0.29	0.40	0.80	0.42
5th to 1st quintile	0.10	0.11	0.34	1.42	0.29

* The figures above show the ratio of the share of each age group in selected quintiles of household income. For example, the value of 0.35 in first cell implies that the share of ISAPRE beneficiaries aged 0-5 in the first income quintile was just over one third of the share of ISAPRE beneficiaries aged 0-5 in the third income quintile.

From self-reported affiliation data from CASEN 90 (Mideplan 1991).

There are concerns that private health insurance does not work efficiently. These concerns centre on the heterogeneity of health plans on offer and the difficulties involved in making reliable evaluations. Larrañaga (1997) reports that in 1995 there were as many as 8,800 different health plans on offer, with different risks covered and different copayment structures. The existing regulations do not require that the ISAPREs provide a minimum or basic health insurance package.

Another important factor explaining health insurance segmentation is the earnings-related mandated contribution. This is grounded on a social insurance principle that has been unwisely extended to private health insurance. Within the social insurance ambit, a mandated earnings-related contribution level best accommodates standard risk pooling

[23] ISAPRE beneficiaries can only access public healthcare on a full cost basis, but due to administrative deficiencies in the latter it was difficult to identify those insured by ISAPREs and recover these costs. An Economic Intelligence Report on Chile notes that 'Cristian Baeza, a former World Bank analyst and FONASA chief until October 1997, estimates that these implicit subsidies to ISAPRE beneficiaries worked out at approximately US$65 million annually' (Economist Intelligence Unit, 1998).

and redistributive objectives. Within a private insurance context, however, it may well produce over- or under-insurance. The mandated level of health contributions may lead to under-insurance by low paid workers and over-insurance by highly paid workers. In the context of health reforms in Chile, it contributes to push high earnings workers towards the ISAPREs and reinforces the observed segmentation. As health insurance contributions are exempt from tax, there is a further incentive for excess demand for health insurance and provision.

Figure 5.3: Health Expenditures as Proportion of GDP, 1976–96

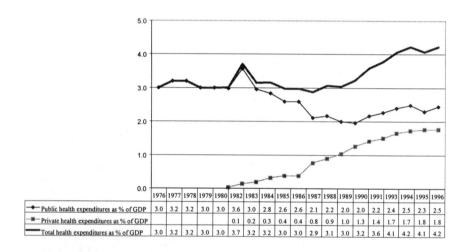

	1976	1977	1978	1979	1980	1982	1983	1984	1985	1986	1987	1988	1989	1990	1991	1993	1994	1995	1996
Public health expenditures as % of GDP	3.0	3.2	3.2	3.0	3.0	3.6	3.0	2.8	2.6	2.6	2.1	2.2	2.0	2.0	2.2	2.4	2.5	2.3	2.5
Private health expenditures as % of GDP						0.1	0.2	0.3	0.4	0.4	0.8	0.9	1.0	1.3	1.4	1.7	1.7	1.8	1.8
Total health expenditures as % of GDP	3.0	3.2	3.2	3.0	3.0	3.7	3.2	3.2	3.0	3.0	2.9	3.1	3.0	3.2	3.6	4.1	4.2	4.1	4.2

Data Sources: Miranda (1994); Larrañaga (1997)

Perhaps the most serious problem emerging from the reforms is that of cost containment in public and private healthcare. Figure 5.3 shows health expenditures as a proportion of GDP, with a strong upward trend in the later period. These figures are an underestimate because over-the-counter pharmacy expenditures and some copayment expenditures are not included. In the private healthcare sector, incentives for cost containment are weak. ISAPREs have in the main restricted themselves to a purchaser role and rely on private healthcare providers who are paid a fee per service, and therefore have little incentive to economise on medical interventions. Individual ISAPRE beneficiaries are required to make a copayment, which should create incentives for cost containment, but their impact is largely negated by the absence of gatekeepers. Chile suffers from a culture of medical 'specialists', so that patients may need to see several specialists and undergo a battery of tests before they find the one relevant to their ailment. Furthermore, in their search for marketing or supply advantage the ISAPREs encourage excess demand for high frequency standard medical interventions.

Incentives for cost containment are also weak within the public health sector. Resource allocation, as noted, was done on a mixture of historic budgets and payment for service. The latter has encouraged an increase in the volume of medical interventions that are covered by the payment for service scheme. In primary care, the government was forced to introduce budgetary caps when faced with a steep rise in interventions. In secondary or tertiary care, copayments for the C and D groups in FONASA can generate incentives for cost containment, but these groups are a minority of all FONASA insured. In 1990, for example, only 18 per cent of FONASA insured belonged to the C and D groups.

The health reforms implemented in the 1980s produced a mixed set of results. The private health insurance sector grew, especially after very supportive legislation and regulatory changes during the early 1980s. It has attracted around a quarter of the population, mostly those with low health risks and high earnings. The expansion of the ISAPREs has generated a strong segmentation in healthcare in Chile. The deterioration of the public healthcare sector as a result of the migration of the better health risk groups to the private sector has reinforced this segmentation in healthcare. The other important policy issue is the rise in health expenditures and the absence of strong cost containment incentives within the public and private healthcare sectors. These were the issues confronting the democratic government, which came to office in 1990.

Modernising public healthcare

The accession to power of a centre-left democratic government in 1990 produced a shift in health policy. Whereas the main focus of health policy in the 1980s was the establishment and development of a private healthcare sector, the new government's focus was on strengthening the public healthcare sector and on reducing inequalities in access to, and quality of, healthcare. The priorities of the democratic government were the improvement in healthcare provision for the more vulnerable sections of the population and the recovery and modernisation of the public healthcare sector. The government also signalled its intention of improving the regulation of the ISAPREs and eliminating cross subsidies from the public to the private healthcare sectors.

Fiscal transfers to the public healthcare sector increased in line with these priorities, from 0.7 per cent of GDP in 1989 to 1.3 per cent in 1996.[24] The extra resources were initially destined to improving the pay of health sector workers and the much-needed refurbishment of hospital facilities, which had deteriorated in the 1980s. By the time the second democratic government took office in 1994, it became apparent that the

[24] Mideplan (1996).

injection of resources into the public healthcare sector had not yielded comparable improvements in service provision. Attention therefore focused on changing incentive structures within the sector to secure administrative and productive efficiency. In 1994 a new capitation funding formula was introduced into primary care and in 1995 a new diagnosis-related payment formula was implemented in the secondary and tertiary care sectors, replacing the existing payment for service funding system.

Primary healthcare

Given the new focus of health policy on improving access and care for the less well off, many new initiatives have been aimed at improving primary care. New Emergency Primary Care Services (Servicios de Atención Primaria de Urgencia — SAPU) have extended primary sector coverage and the deployment of 'third shifts' in primary care units helped to extend opening times. The new Primary Healthcare Worker Statute (Estatuto de Atención Primaria Municipal) approved in 1995 lays down conditions of service, and career structures, for health professionals in this sector.

A key innovation has been the introduction of capitation funding for primary care institutions. This began to be implemented in 1994 and replaces the payment for service (Facturación por Atenciones Prestadas en Establecimientos Municipales — FAPEM) funding formula in place since the early 1980s. This had been subject to budget caps, which distorted its function and contributed to inequalities in provision across municipalities.[25] The new capitation funding formula is based on the costing of a Family Health Plan (Plan de Salud Familiar), including a basic basket of health interventions, which is adjusted for demographic and epidemiological variations.[26] The new capitation funding formula has also encouraged the registration of patients, which should improve administrative controls, encourage participation and eliminate cross subsidies to ISAPREs and other private beneficiaries.[27]

Secondary and tertiary healthcare

A key objective in the improvement of secondary and tertiary public healthcare has been a programme of capital and equipment investment in hospitals[28] and the reduction of waiting lists. Although the structure of the public healthcare sector has remained largely intact, some changes were introduced. These include the establishment of a regulator for the ISAPREs (the Superintendencia de ISAPREs) in 1990, a function which had previously been performed by FONASA.

---

[25] Duarte (1995)

[26] Fuenzalida (1995) remarks on the fact that this was the first time a basic package of healthcare had been defined in Chile.

[27] Primary care is free to FONASA insured and ISAPRE beneficiaries cannot register with public primary care units.

[28] Mideplan (1996).

A new funding formula for secondary and tertiary healthcare was introduced, with the diagnosis-related payment formula replacing in 1995 the payment for service formula (FAP). As noted, the payment for service formula had limited impact, further restricted by the absence of reliable service costing or 'prices'. The payment for service formula, to the extent that it had an impact, encouraged units to increase the volume of measured interventions, without reference to outcomes.[29] The need to generate greater incentives for service efficiency within the public healthcare sector led to the introduction of diagnosis-related payments. It defined a set of standard interventions associated with each diagnosis or group of diagnoses, which are later valued at average service costs for a sample of health units. This funding method provides incentives for units with lower than average cost to provide more services and makes it less economical for units with above average cost to provide the service. The diagnosis-related payment is expected to cover between 40 and 50 per cent of inpatient expenditures.[30] In cases where there is no defined diagnosis, or where complications arise, the funding is set according to a prospective payment-for-service formula.[31] The new funding formulas are expected to provide strong incentives for micro-efficiency and cost containment. They have coincided with the introduction of computerised administrative and registration systems which should reduce or eliminate cross subsidies to the private healthcare sector.

Decentralisation of public health services

A major emphasis of health policy has been placed on the decentralisation of public services. Decentralisation is defined by the government as the process of 'transferring resources, risks and opportunities to the Health Services (Servicios de Salud)'.[32] It is the intention of the government to extend decentralisation to cover the contracting and management of labour resources, as well as other services or inputs; and the deployment of resources and services to meet local needs. This is likely to be strongly opposed by health unions concerned with the erosion of collective bargaining and national conditions of service and pay. The new funding formulas discussed above fit in well with this strategy.

The ISAPREs

The modernisation of the public healthcare system will, in itself, put pressure on the ISAPREs to improve their performance. The democratic government's health policy has aimed to eliminate the large cross subsidies from the public healthcare sector to the private one, which had been allowed to develop in the 1980s. Although the ISAPRE beneficiaries are not entitled to seek medical care from the public health institutions, a 1992

---

[29] Lenz (1995).

[30] *Ibid.*

[31] In the case of more complex procedures, funding is negotiated between the Ministry of Health and the relevant specialised units (Rodríguez, 1995).

[32] Ministerio de Salud (1998b).

household survey indicated that large numbers of them had. The survey indicated that the proportion of ISAPRE beneficiaries having received healthcare from public health institutions stood at 30 per cent in the case of preventive medicine, 39 per cent in the case of hospitalisations, and 69 per cent in the case of emergencies. Moreover, 42 per cent of childbirth to ISAPRE beneficiaries had been performed in public hospitals.[33] The new administrative procedures and the computerisation of registers in the public sector will make it very difficult for ISAPRE beneficiaries to seek healthcare from public health sector institutions, both in the primary care sector and the secondary and tertiary care sector.

The government has also taken steps to eliminate the extra two per cent subsidy to low income workers joining the ISAPREs and has sought to regulate the ISAPREs to achieve greater transparency and comparability in the health plans on offer and in healthcare contracts. It has also taken the ISAPREs to task for their lack of coverage of the older population.

In sum, the return to democracy has been accompanied by a more inclusive health policy, with greater emphasis on extending access and improving services for the more vulnerable sections of the population. This has resulted in a recovery of the public healthcare sector, which has been better resourced and modernised. Health policy has also attempted to eliminate cross subsidies to the private healthcare sector and to focus resources on primary care.

Problems and challenges

The ebbs and flows of health policy have left a number of important problems and issues unresolved and created a few new ones. This section discusses some of the main problems and challenges for health policy in Chile.

The private and public healthcare sectors: complements or substitutes?

The expansion of the private health sector in the 1980s and the recovery of the public health sector in the 1990s have not yet resolved the issue of how these sectors should best be articulated. The question is whether they ought to be in competition with one another, or whether they should be integrated in some way. In order to address this issue it is necessary to distinguish between private health provision and private health insurance. The provision of private healthcare predated the 1980 health reform for white-collar workers. There is a measure of consensus in the view that it is both useful and desirable that private healthcare provision be integrated within an all-embracing healthcare system, preferably as a complement to existing public provision. In the context of the current situation in Chile, this principle would suggest the possibility of allowing the ISAPREs to negotiate the use of public healthcare facilities, which is at present allowed only in exceptional circumstances.[34]

---

[33] Mideplan (1996).
[34] This could help to increase public healthcare sector utilisation and revenues and perhaps fa-

The issue of how to integrate private health insurance is more complex. At present, the private health insurance providers compete with social health insurance. This competition is sui generis since FONASA is the 'insurer of last resort'. ISAPREs negotiate individual health plans with their affiliates, which restrict the risks covered, establish ceilings for claims and specify copayment levels. The outcome of the individual contract is to limit the range of insurance provided by the ISAPREs. Moreover, it is likely that these restrictions help the ISAPREs discriminate between the good and bad health risk groups and to attract the former. By contrast, the range of insurance provided by FONASA is limited only by resource policy for public healthcare provision and by regulation for the use of private providers. The range of insurance provided by FONASA is wider and more open-ended than that provided by the ISAPREs.

As ISAPRE beneficiaries can at any time return to FONASA, they can rely on this broader insurance of last resort. They return to FONASA, for example, when their health risk deteriorates through age or catastrophic illness. Kifmann (1998) argues that for a significant group of ISAPRE beneficiaries, affiliation amounts to accessing insurance for outpatient care, which is additional to the inpatient care provided by public insurance. Characterised in this way, ISAPREs only provide additional health insurance (insurance for outpatient services), while the public health insurance scheme provides full insurance.

This articulation of private and social health insurance has a number of drawbacks. Migrating to the ISAPREs improves the welfare of those able to do so, but it reduces overall welfare. This is because the capacity of the public health insurance sector to provide actuarially sound insurance declines as the better health groups migrate to the ISAPREs, only to return once their health risk status deteriorates. This particular form of competition therefore leads to a number of undesirable outcomes. The situation would be different if the option to switch back to the public health insurance scheme was withdrawn, as this would force the ISAPREs to provide life-cycle health insurance, rather than short-term annual contracts. It would also call attention to the need to introduce some form of risk adjustment within the ISAPRE sector to preclude self-selection, as has been the case with private health providers in most developed countries.[35]

In sum, health policy should strive to create the conditions under which the private and public healthcare sectors are fully complementary in healthcare provision. However, as regards insurance their current articulation has not proved successful. There are conditions under which complementarity between the private and public sector health insurance is feasible. These would require distinguishing between a basic mandatory health insurance package, provided mainly by the public health insurance fund, and

cilitate cost containment within the private healthcare sector (Caviedes, 1996).
[35] Oxley and MacFarlan (1994).

voluntary additional health insurance perhaps to be provided mainly by private health insurance funds. It is not clear if this is an option in Chile.

Studies of the Chilean private health insurance market have concluded that information costs preclude the market from delivering expected efficiency gains.[36] The bewildering variety of health plans on offer allied to their opaqueness makes it impossible for consumers to compare and evaluate them. In part this is a consequence of the mandated level of health contributions, which encourages health plan differentiation. One possible solution is to regulate for the construction of reliable comparators, a strategy the government has attempted in recent legislation. The problems associated with information costs and asymmetries are well known in insurance markets and justify a measure of scepticism on the chances of finding effective solutions. The information asymmetries existing between patients and health professionals generate conventional problems of supplier-induced demand and micro-inefficiency. Within the public healthcare sector the separation of purchasers and providers within the health system emerges as a possible solution. In the context of Chile, this separation could be brought about by enlarging the role of FONASA to act as an active and effective purchaser of healthcare. An enlarged role for FONASA was considered in the 1994 strategic reform plan for the public healthcare sector,[37] but has not materialised. This would require that FONASA takes an active role in negotiating services from providers on behalf of those it insured, as well as in providing information to guide the choices of beneficiaries.

Cost containment of health expenditures

In common with a number of countries at a similar stage of development, Chile's health expenditures show a rising trend. This trend has been marked in the late 1980s and '90s, in part as a result of the rise in fiscal transfers to the public healthcare sector since 1990, but also as a direct result of the lack of cost containment incentives within the private healthcare sector. In the public sector it is expected that the new funding formulas in place will facilitate cost containment.

However, the US experience shows that diagnosis-related financing is not without its dangers.[38] These include a potential incentive to discharge patients prematurely (where this does not alter the value of the lump sum paid for the diagnosis) and the problem of 'diagnosis creep' (where practitioners will provide the most expensive diagnosis, whenever possible). Clearly, this form of financing relies heavily on the competence and integrity of the health professionals responsible for diagnosis. In the private healthcare sector this is more difficult to achieve, partly due to the strong and persistent marketing pressures on the ISAPREs, but also because these have largely restricted themselves to a purchaser role. Cost containment in the private healthcare sector sug-

---

[36] Kifmann (1998); Miranda et al. (1995); and Oyarzo (1994).
[37] Oyarzo and Galleguillos (1995).
[38] Able-Smith (1994).

gests some form of vertical integration with these providers as a means of controlling service costs, as has been the experience with Health Maintenance Organisations in the USA.

Conclusions

This chapter has outlined the changes in health policy experienced in Chile in recent decades. In the 1950s and '60s Chile developed a centralised public healthcare system, financed through social insurance contributions and fiscal transfers. In 1980 a radical change in health policy aimed at enlarging the scope for private health insurance and provision. The creation of the ISAPREs in 1980 and their subsequent development extended private sector involvement in healthcare to the area of health insurance. The public healthcare sector deteriorated in the 1980s in part as a result of fiscal entrenchment and in part to encourage migration of workers to the ISAPREs. The democratic government shifted health policy again towards the reconstruction and modernisation of the public healthcare sector.

Currently, around a quarter of the population is affiliated to the private health insurance funds, the ISAPREs, with a further two thirds covered by the public health insurance fund, FONASA. The 1980s health reforms resulted in a strong segmentation of health insurance, with the better health risk, and higher income, groups migrating to the ISAPREs. FONASA retained the responsibility to finance healthcare for inactive and non-insured groups. This segmentation undermined the capacity of the public health insurance fund to finance adequate health provision for the majority of the population. The 1990s change in health policy has sought to restore the public healthcare sector's capacity to satisfy the healthcare needs of the majority of the population and especially those of the less well off.

The next decade will show whether this strategy is successful. Its success will depend on its meeting the challenges posed by some key unresolved problems arising from the successive changes in health policy. These include the search for a better articulation of private and private health insurance; the need to complete the modernisation of the public healthcare sector and the need to strengthen cost containment mechanisms in health expenditure.

CHAPTER 6

Health System Reforms in Cuba in the 1990s

Richard Garfield and Timothy H. Holtz

Introduction

Since the 1960s, health sector investments in Cuba have been made via a strong public sector also dedicated to equitable food distribution, public education and income equalisation.[1] Enviable health and medical care indicators were produced by this system despite the US embargo. In the 1990s, the combined effect of severe economic decline and a far more stringent embargo have severely tested the capacity and flexibility of that system. In 1990 Cuba adopted a range of emergency measures, known as the 'special period in time of peace'. These saw the introduction of near-total food rationing and strict controls on the use of oil and petroleum.[2] Equitable distribution of scarce goods and priority programmes for vulnerable populations help explain the apparent contradiction between a massive decline in available resources, a deteriorating public health infrastructure and rising incidence rates for infectious diseases and low birth weight, on the one hand, and continued low rates of infant mortality, on the other.

Health system 'reforms' have occurred throughout the developing world in the 1990s. Most of these reforms aim to privatise curative services, raise funds through subscription and user fees and make public services more efficient. Ironically, reduced public funding for curative services and the primacy of financial institutions (for example, the World Bank) over technical ones (for example, the World Health Organisation) in leading the reform has occurred together with a rhetorical emphasis on human development and investing in the health and wellbeing of populations in poor countries.[3]

Cuba has the lowest infant and maternal mortality rates, the highest doctor-to-population ratio and the highest rate of public health service coverage in Latin America.[4] Its national health system, like its political and social systems, is not participating in the global trend toward privatisation of essential goods and human services. Yet Cuba faces similar economic pressures to the market economies, particularly since it lost trade and aid relations with the Soviet Union in 1991 and the subsequent US tightening of its economic embargo in 1992.[5] Despite its apparent stability, the Cuban health system is undergoing major changes and will face more in the near

---

[1] Based in part on Garfield and Santana (1997), pp. 15–20.
[2] Cole (1998).
[3] World Bank (1993a).
[4] Pan American Health Organisation (1995a).
[5] Feinsilver (1993).

future. Here we analyse these changes and identify policy alternatives available to the healthcare system.

Health continues to receive high and rising budget allocations in an attempt to preserve the main gains of socialism. In health, these include:[6]

- Universal coverage

- An excellent information and research structure to support public health

- Extensive primary care services, including a widespread family doctor programme

- Targeted activities to deal with the special health needs of women, children and workers

- Cradle-to-grave benefits which, in better times, were among the most generous in the world

- An advanced biomedical research and product industry

The essential principles of the system, as summarised in a planning document in 1997,[7] are:

- To maintain coverage and access to health services without user fees

- To finance all health services exclusively by the state

The medical system is still able to provide near universal coverage and to ensure the continuance of low mortality among those under 65 years of age, even in the face of rising health threats. Yet, despite the highly efficient use of health goods, these goods can no longer be stretched to meet the needs of the entire population. Preferential access to essential goods for women and children is exemplary but has resulted in the creation of new vulnerable groups among adult men and the elderly.

Background

The US embargo against Cuba began in 1961, following the 1959 Cuban Revolution. At that time, it had a limited impact because of Soviet assistance and egalitarian distribution policies. During the following three decades, 70 to 90 per cent of Cuba's international trade was with the former Soviet bloc,[8] and health and other social indices improved dramatically.

From 1965 to 1975, the economy grew at an annual rate of about two per cent. Starting in 1975, the embargo was modified to permit trade with US subsidiary firms in other countries during the period of cold war détente. From 1975 to 1989, the economy grew at an annual rate of about four per cent. Dissolution of the Soviet Union and the

---

[6] MINSAP (1997).

[7] Eckstein (1997).

[8] D. Vallinas, Cuban vice-minister of economics, personal communication (February 1994).

COMECON (Community for Economic Cooperation) trade group in 1989 greatly weakened the Cuban economy. Soviet Bloc exports to Cuba declined by about 70 per cent from 1989 to 1993, the gross national product (GNP) declined by 35 per cent and the value of imports from all sources declined from US$8 billion to US$1.7 billion.[9]

In 1992 the US embargo was made more stringent with the passage of the Cuban Democracy Act. All US subsidiary trade, including trade in food and medicines, has since been prohibited. Ships from other countries are not allowed to dock at US ports for six months after visiting Cuba, even if their cargoes are humanitarian goods. Pressure is being applied on other countries to stop trading with, or providing humanitarian goods to, Cuba. Although embargo legislation since World War II has usually included exemptions for humanitarian goods, the 1992 embargo legislation on Cuba does not permit sales of food and requires unprecedented 'on-site verification' for the donation of medical supplies.[10] The legislation does not state that Cuba cannot purchase medicines from US companies or their foreign subsidiaries; however, such license requests have often been delayed or denied.

The embargo's effects on nutrition

About half of all protein and calories intended for human consumption were imported by Cuba in the 1980s. Importation of foodstuffs declined by about 50 per cent from 1989 to 1993 and per capita protein and calorie availability from all sources declined by 25 per cent and 18 per cent, respectively, from 1989 to 1992. Only about 1,200 calories a day are available from low-cost rationed distribution. The shortage of calories is exacerbated by the high proportion of all calories from refined sugar, which increased from 18 per cent in 1989 to 26 per cent in 1992.

The nutritional situation continued to decline until unrestricted agricultural markets opened in late 1994. This private sector is estimated to provide about a ten per cent caloric supplement to the population. Children, women and the elderly have been targeted for protection from nutritional deficits through rationing, public health education, workplace and school-based feeding programmes and the promotion of urban gardening. As a result, sentinel site data show that the burden of calorie, protein and micronutrient deficits falls predominately on adult men (Figure 6.1), whose caloric intake fell from 3,100 in 1989 to 1,863 in 1994.

The proportion of newborns weighing under 2,500g rose by 23 per cent, from 7.3 per cent in 1989 to 9.0 per cent in 1993, reversing ten years of gradual progress (Figure 6.2). Virtually all of the country's 150,000 annual births occur in health institutions, which is in sharp contrast with most other countries in the region. The fall in birthweights

---

[9] From press conference given by Carlos Lage, vice president of the Council of State, International Press Centre, Havana, 23 July 1996.

[10] Kirkpatrick (1996).

occurred despite a decline in other risk factors for low birthweight, including smoking, high fertility and births to women under the age of 20. Presumably the rate of low birthweights would have risen far more if preferential rationing and supplemental food programmes were not in place. However, although enrolment in supplemental feeding programmes at maternity centres tripled from 1989 to 1992, food was still lacking and weight gains remained poor. Moreover, the ability to provide such supplements has been declining. Guaranteed daily milk rations previously reached all children up to and including age 13 and all those over the age of 65. Since 1992, however, these rations have been provided only to children up to the age of seven. More foods are now being procured by sending women to eat at nearby workers' cafeterias, setting aside milk and eggs from nearby state farms, and generating dollar donations from workers in tourist industries.

Figure 6.1: Nutrition Levels Relative to Recommended Minimum by Age and Sex, 1992

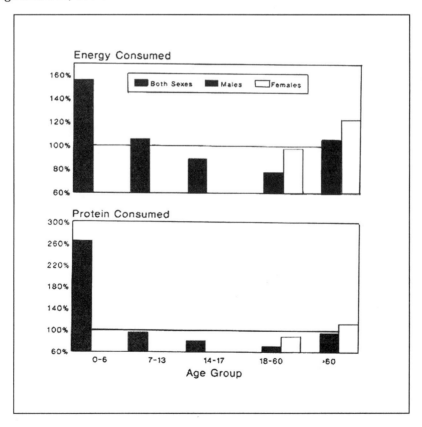

Data Source: Ministry of Public Health (MINSAP), Anuario Estadístico.

Data on weight and weight gain among pregnant women are routinely collected by clinicians and analysed by provincial Ministry of Public Health authorities. From 1988 to 1993, the percentage of women with inadequate weight at pregnancy rose by 18 per cent, from 7.9 per cent to 9.3 per cent and that of women with weight gains of less than eight kilograms during pregnancy rose from 5.3 per cent to 5.8 per cent. Anaemia affected more than 50 per cent of pregnant women and infants from six to 12 months of age in 1991. Rates of anaemia this high had not been seen since survey data were first collected in the early 1970s.[11]

Figure 6.2: Low Weight Births in Cuba, 1980–96

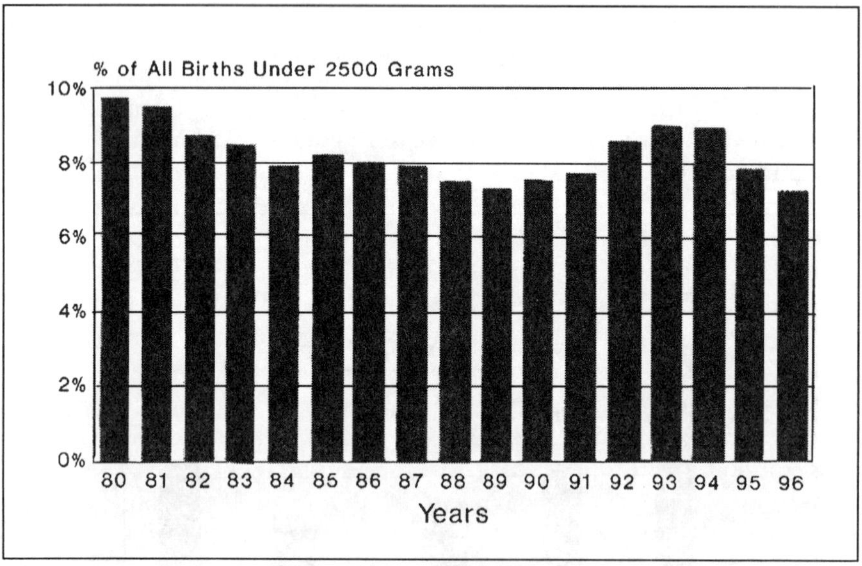

Data Source: Ministry of Public Health (MINSAP).

Undernutrition is the major risk factor associated with an epidemic of optic neuropathy, which has affected more than 51,000 people since 1992. Since late 1992, the entire population has been provided with monthly vitamin supplements to protect against this disorder. These vitamins are distributed door to door by family physicians. The few new cases diagnosed each month occur predominantly among those who fail to take the supplements.

Cuba's public health infrastructure and medical outcomes

Cuba's economic decline in the 1990s has been associated with a reduction in the materials and products needed to ensure clean water. From 1990 to 1994, the proportion of the population with domestic water connections de-

---

[11] John Guy, personal communication (July 1995).

clined for the first time, from 83 to 81 per cent in urban areas and from 30 to 24 per cent in rural areas. During the same period, the portion of the population without access to potable water increased from ten to 12 per cent. The country's ability to produce chlorine declined, reducing the population covered by chlorinated water systems from 98 per cent in 1988 to 26 per cent in 1994. During the first week of July 1994, only 13 per cent of the country's 161 municipal water systems were chlorinated. Mortality from diarrhoeal diseases per 100,000 population rose from 2.7 in 1989 to 6.8 in 1993. International donations and imports subsequently made up for the deficit in chlorine production so that during the first week of July 1995, 87 per cent of the municipal water systems were chlorinated.

Poor nutrition and deteriorating housing and sanitary conditions are as-sociated with a rising incidence of tuberculosis, from 5.5 per 100,000 in 1990 to 15.3 per 100,000 in 1994. Cuba had a serious housing shortage in the 1980s and has built virtually no residential housing since. Consequently, 15 per cent of the country's housing stock is in poor condition, including 1,000 homes that collapsed in Havana in 1994 and 4,000 more that are in a precarious state today. Medication shortages were associated with a 48 per cent increase in tuberculosis deaths from 1992 to 1993. And from 1989 to 1993, these conditions were also associated with a 67 per cent increase in deaths due to infections and parasitic diseases (from 8.3 to 13.9 per 100,000 population) and a 77 per cent increase in deaths due to influenza and pneumonia (from 23.0 to 40.7 per 100,000 population, see Figure 6.3).

Lack of fats formerly imported from the Soviet Union resulted in a severe shortage in soap and soap products. Yearly per capita soap dis-tributed via rationing in 1993 and '94 amounted to four small bars. Soap substitutes are made with caustic soda and other chemicals not normally found in the home. These chemicals cause burns and poisonings, which were extremely rare before 1989. From 1989 to 1993, deaths from un-intentional poisonings jumped from 0.4 to 1.1 per 100,000 population. During the week of 13 June 1994, six cases of unintended oesophageal burns were reported to the epidemiological surveillance system. Three of these were caused by caustic soda; the other three were caused by kerosene, which is commonly used to light homes during electricity blackouts. Inability to procure appropriate receptacles and the lack of appropriate labelling for home-made products both contribute to this problem. In November 1994, a large stock of homemade soap was sold throughout Pinar del Rio province in used rum bottles. Within a week, five cases of oesophageal burns resulted from its accidental ingestion and the Ministry of Public Health recalled the product.

Reductions in public transportation and employment have affected the country's morbidity profile. Motor vehicle-related deaths declined by 28 per cent while bicycle-related deaths rose by 78 per cent from 1989 to 1993. An increase in small-scale, unsupervised agricultural and indus-trial production is responsible for new occupational exposures.

Figure 6.3: Deaths from Infectious and Parasitic Diseases, 1985–1996

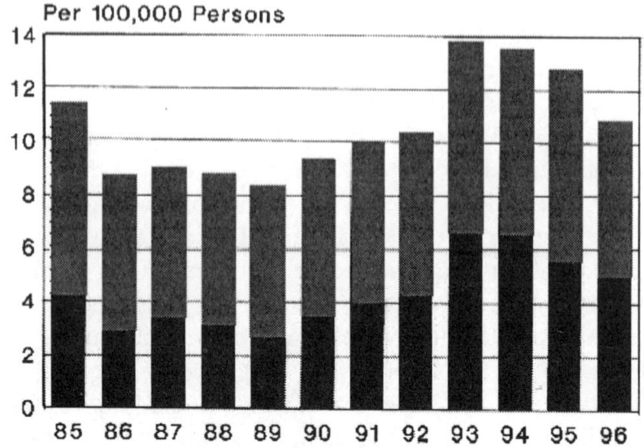

	85	86	87	88	89	90	91	92	93	94	95	96
Other Inf/Para	7.1	5.8	5.6	5.7	5.6	5.9	5.9	6.2	7.2	7	7.3	5.8
Acute Diarrhoea	4.3	2.9	3.4	3.1	2.7	3.5	4	4.2	6.6	6.5	5.5	5

Data Source: Ministry of Public Health (MINSAP)

Total mortality per 1,000 inhabitants rose from 6.4 in 1989 to 7.2 in 1994. The increase was almost entirely due to a 15 per cent rise in mortality among those aged 65 years and over, accounting for 7,500 excess deaths (see Figure 6.4). From 1992 to 1993 alone, the death rate for influenza and pneumonia, tuberculosis, diarrhoea, suicide, unintentional injuries, asthma and heart disease each rose by at least ten per cent among this older population. In all other age groups, mortality rates remained stable or declined.

By 1994, however, deteriorating social conditions and medical facilities began to affect other population groups as well. Infant mortality rose slightly, owing to an increase in deaths caused by respiratory and diarrhoeal diseases. A rise in the maternal mortality rate in 1994 and '95 is associated with declining maternal nutritional status, untreated vaginal infections and shortages in parts for transportation and electricity during emergency deliveries. Both infant and maternal mortality reached their lowest level ever during the first six months of 1996.

Social disruption caused by declining public transportation, lack of repairs, rising unemployment and underemployment and economic instability are widely perceived as reducing the quality of urban life. Partially protected are the 21 per cent of Cubans estimated to have access to domestic dollar incomes or to receive remittances from family overseas. The disappearance of begging, prostitution, homelessness and children without shoes in the 1960s had often been described as 'achievements of the revolution' in years past. The reappearance of these phenomena is now being observed in major cities.

Figure 6.4: Mortality among Selected Groups, 1984–90

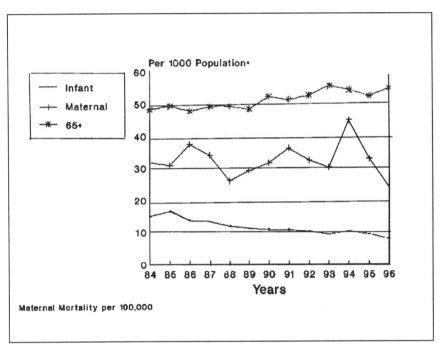

Data Source: Ministry of Public Health (MINSAP)

Yet despite severe resource shortages, immunisation coverage among children under two years of age is still higher than 90 per cent. No cases of measles have been reported since 1993. In 1993, the World Health Organisation certified Cuba as the first country to be free of the circulation of wild polio virus.

Health services

Continuing high educational levels, a national system of nutritional monitoring and ready access to health services are key to protecting the population. Per capita funding for the health system rose each year since the 1960s until 1990, when it declined slightly. It rose again starting in 1993, in part as a result of the additional costs associated with the country's optic neuropathy epidemic. However, while per capita funding was valued at about US$150 during the 1980s, high inflation since 1990 has drastically reduced the value of these funds.

The number of hospital beds per capita is stable, and the high rate of physicians per capita continues to rise (see Figure 6.5). Family medicine specialists practising in the local communities now serve more than 90 per cent of the population. The physician per population ratio has risen steadily during the last 25 years.

Figure 6.5: Physicians and Beds in Cuba per 100,000 Population, 1984–96

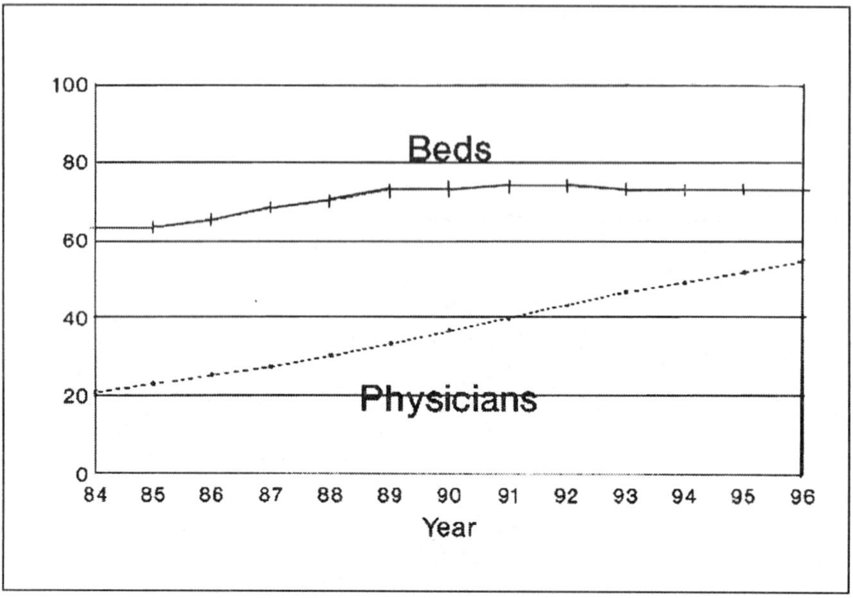

Data Source: Ministry of Public Health (MINSAP)

From 1990 to 1994, the number of laboratory exams provided in the country's 273 hospitals declined by 36 per cent and the number of X rays declined by 75 per cent. Cuba used to have an accessible national formulary of 1,300 products; in recent years this was reduced to 889 and at least a third of these products is now unavailable at any given time. Ambulance access has become scarce, as spare parts are increasingly difficult to obtain. Most ambulances were in working order in the 1980s; fewer than half worked in June 1994.

Minimising the impact of the embargo and the economic crisis on vulnerable groups

Cuba's approach to the economic crisis has been based on the dual policies of equity and priority for vulnerable groups. The government was already skilled at rationing food and other scarce goods prior to 1989. It has since used the mass media and workplaces to promote the use of bicycles in place of cars, animals in place of tractors and trucks (for which fuel and parts are lacking) and the consumption of vegetable-based foods in place of scarce animal protein. In hospitals, rooming-in and other baby-friendly changes have sought to promote exclusive breast-feeding further. Eighty per cent of all births now occur in such baby-friendly hospitals, and the prevalence of breast-feeding at the time of postpartum discharge has risen from 63 per cent in 1990 to 97 per cent in 1994. Clinics, hospitals and day care centres have helped to popularise the use of herbal medicines to replace scarce pharmaceuticals. Distribution of food, clothing and other scarce goods to target groups, including women, the elderly and children, is facilitated via social service institutions, workplaces, pre-schools and maternity homes. The number of children in pre-schools doubled and the use of maternity homes among those waiting to give birth rose by 26 per cent from 1988 to 1993.

Table 6.1: Health Spending in Cuba, 1989–96

Year	Peso health spending (millions)	Peso health spending per capita	Spending as per cent of GNP	Spending as per cent of total govt. budget
1989	1,023	97	4.6	5.8
1990	1,045	99	4.7	6.0
1991	1,039	97	5.4	6.3
1992	1,040	96	6.2	6.6
1993	1,176	108	8.4	7.4
1994	1,166	106	8.2	7.5
1995	1,222	111	8.4	8.0
1996	1,310	119	8.6	9.6

Source: MINSAP (1997).

Health sector finance

Throughout 1997, the Ministry of Health (MINSAP) continued to receive high and stable budgetary allocations from the government (see Table 6.1). At the beginning of the special period it was thought that the health system would lose up to 30 per cent of its funds. In fact, the emergence of an epidemic of optic neuropathy in 1991 and subsequent attempt to expand the safety net of public services resulted in increased spending for the health system. *Peso* budgets, however, obscure a serious decline in the purchasing power of these funds. Before the special period, the *peso* was pegged at a fixed exchange rate of one to the dollar. During 1992 the black market value of the *peso* fell to 120 to the dollar; by 1997 it had recovered to 22 to the dollar. Loss of purchasing power of the *peso* gutted salaries and decimated ministry budgets. Its main impact was to make imports, such as medicines and spare parts, far more expensive. By 1992 the curative health system began to look like an empty shell of its former self, with ample buildings and personnel but almost without equipment or medicines with which to work.[12]

Public spending on the health sector consumed about 8.6 per cent of the gross national product by 1996.[13] This was about twice the proportion of the GNP consumed by the health sector at the beginning of the decade and a higher proportion than public spending in any other country in the hemisphere. (The closest was Costa Rica at 6.9 per cent, followed by the Argentina at 5.3 per cent and the US at 5.1 per cent).[14] This figure does not include all aspects of the health system such as construction, research and development and training. It also undervalues the importance of imports, a particularly important input in countries with poor rates of exchange.

Figure 6.6: Medical Supplies Imported in US Dollars, 1989–96

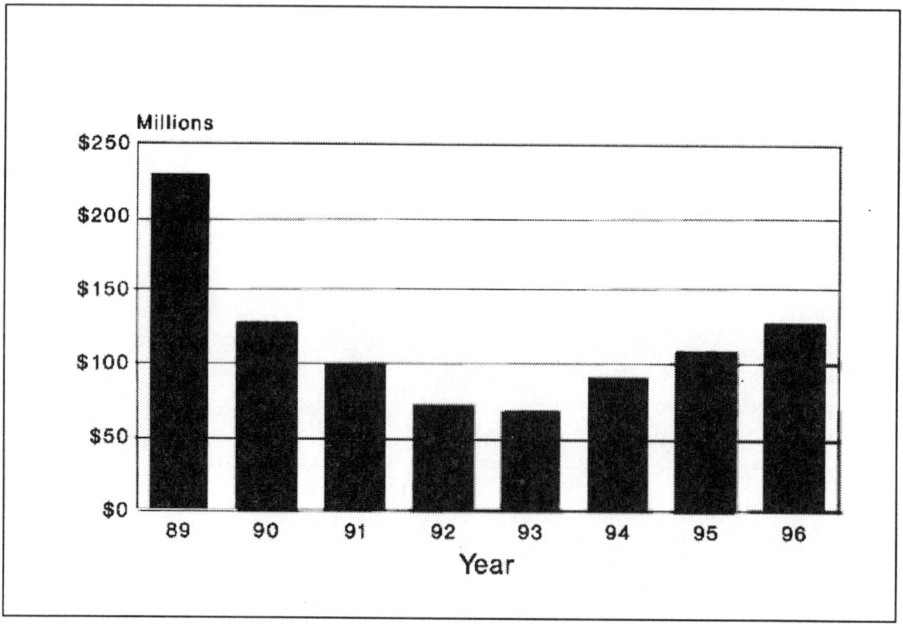

Data Source: Ministry of Public Health (MINSAP).

Changes in the value of goods imported for the health system more closely mirror the economic fortunes of the country. In 1989 Cuba imported US$227 million in health related goods (see Figure 6.6). Part of this value was in-kind or exchange goods as part of COMECON con-

---

[12] French (1993).
[13] Departamento de Planificación (1997).
[14] Pan American Health Organisation (1995a).

tracts. These non-monetary estimates disappeared after 1989 with the loss of these socialist trade relations. By 1993 this value had fallen by about 70 per cent, to US$67 million. Subsequent modest economic recovery led to imports of US$127 million in health goods in 1996, still 40 per cent lower than 1989. Yet even these reduced dollar inputs were worth double all the *peso* inputs to the system at then-current black market rates of exchange.

Economic reforms

Economic limitations in the special period dictated that only some programmes could be preserved. The most dramatic change was legalising the de facto dollarisation of the economy. Goods as basic as cooking oil, salt and many medicines in the early 1990s could only be purchased in dollars. Private enterprise, employment in the tourist sector or remittances from family members living outside Cuba used to be treated with suspicion or worse. Now some of these non-socialist activities would be tolerated and legalised. About 15 per cent of those employed earn some dollars and another 21 per cent are estimated to receive remittances from family members in other countries.[15] In all, close to half of families have direct access to dollars. Under the watchful eye of the Communist Party and with heavy taxation and regulation, markets re-emerged in Cuba, foreign firms invested and an entrepreneurial class of Cubans emerged in the 1990s.

Under socialism, everyone was guaranteed a job. Hidden unemployment in duplicative or grossly unproductive activities usually did not exceed ten per cent of the population. By 1995, about 45 per cent of the economically active population was de facto unemployed. New jobs now exist almost exclusively in the small-scale private service sector of 110 legalised fields of self-employment or via employment by a foreign firm. By 1996 225 foreign companies signed contracts to provide US$2 billion to reactivate the Cuban economy, at a profit. The state used to directly control more than 95 per cent of all economic activity. It now probably accounts directly for around half.

Rationed goods sold at heavily subsidised prices in the 1960s and 1970s provided for nearly all basic needs. Abundance of food and other basic goods by the 1980s reduced the need for the ration, and about half of all basic goods were sold off the ration. The role of the ration has changed again in the special period. Although food and other essentials are scarce, the ration now provides for less than half of essential goods and it is not always available. For the first time since the Cuban Revolution in 1959, some people have ample money and do not seek rationed goods, while others depend on the ration more than ever. Although calories available from the ration are down, private agricultural markets are associated with a rise in average calorie consumption as well as a rise in inequality of calorie distribution.

---

[15] Pan American Health Organisation (1996).

The health system has been modified to respond to these changes in several ways. First, a tax system has been established to take in resources from the private sector, in order to fund public goods, including health. A recent policy document on health finance stated, 'As a result of the necessary measures to adapt our economy to the real world, some sectors (of the population) have higher incomes than the rest. Social services will not be used to … introduce deformities and privileges that are incompatible with the principles [of the revolution] … This is the place for the tax system, so that he who has more income provides more to the finance of the state.'[16] In 1997, the private sector made up 2.5 per cent of the gross domestic product (GDP) and 4.5 per cent of state revenues.[17]

A second source of new funding for health is domestic and international donations. Outside the tax system, appeals to workers in privileged sectors have resulted in millions of *pesos* worth of donations. Union members pool tips and make monthly decisions about their distribution to each worker and donations outside their sector. The Hotel and Tourism Worker's Union provided US$882,000 to MINSAP in 1996 and US$1 million in 1997. Sometimes profitable state or private firms also adopt a particular hospital or school to provide ongoing support to a cancer ward, to provide cleaning supplies or to provide goods for birthday parties for hospitalised children.

In the 1970s and '80s Cuba provided extensive international assistance via direct domestic health services, training of foreign doctors and medical teams sent overseas. This international assistance was worth at least ten per cent of the health budget, or an estimated US$50 million per year. Cuba was so active in medical assistance that it was scarcely observed that there was little direct health assistance to Cuba from other countries or international organisations. With the tightening of the US embargo in 1992, MINSAP set up an office to facilitate the receipt of international donations. By the late 1990s about US$20 million in value was received each year as international donations. About US$5 million came from UN related organisations, US$10 million in donation of goods from solidarity and religious groups in the US and Europe, governments and non-governmental organisations (US$7 million worth of medicines, US$3 million worth of other medical supplies).[18] At this level, international assistance provided for nine per cent of dollar health spending in 1994. Another US$5 million in unregistered donations may go directly to hospitals and clinics.

Cuba also developed a market for its health services and products in response to the special period. Investment in biomedical products was the third largest investment area for the economy in the early 1990s. MEDICUBA sells 20 biomedical products internationally. It generated an income of US$135 million from these products in 1997.[19] There is now one

---

[16] Departamento de Planificación (1997).

[17] MINSAP (1997).

[18] Personal communication, Enrique Comandero, director of the Office of Donations, MINSAP, 18 Aug. 1997.

[19] MINSAP (1997).

hospital designated exclusively for foreigners who pay in dollars. It provided care to 1,218 Europeans and 92 US citizens in 1996. Many leading hospitals also have some wards or beds available for payment in dollars. Also, the Cuban government keeps 30 per cent of the income of doctors under contract overseas. Together, these entrepreneurial sources accounted for 13 per cent of dollar income for MINSAP in 1994.

The largest source of dollars for health imports, about 75 per cent or US$60 million in 1994, was provided by central government allocations. In order to protect these funds from international creditors, the Cuban government created an innovative arrangement to transfer funds directly from dollar-generating ministries to MINSAP without passing through the central budget coffers.

Of the *peso* funds used to run the health system, 88 per cent of allocations came from funds administered by local government bodies in 1996. Like most developing countries, the Cuban health system in the 1980s, with an extensive network of modern hospitals, spent about half of all health funds in hospitals. The most advanced research hospital in the country alone consumed about ten per cent of the country's health budget. The inability of the health system to maintain all aspects of specialist care during the special period, combined with the rapid growth of the family doctor system, led to a shift in favour of primary care. Primary care received about a third of the health budget in the 1980s, by the mid-1990s this had grown to half. Overall, from 1985–94 the proportion of the health budget going to hospitals fell by 18 per cent, the proportion going to medicines rose by 33 per cent and the proportion going to ambulatory care rose by 55 per cent.[20]

Weaknesses in the health system

Delayed maintenance of hospitals and a dramatic reduction in availability of medicines resulted in a loss in the ability to provide high quality specialist care in the 1990s. By the early 1990s, the family doctor system should have led to a reduced frequency of hospitalisations, shorter hospital stays and a decline in the bed-to-population ratio. Ironically, weakening of the hospital system resulted in more, and relatively longer, hospital stays. Cost savings and care innovations were few. In 1996, when a new network of ambulances was put into operation, physicians even hesitated to transfer patients from the ambulances into emergency departments and intensive care units because they were more poorly equipped. In 1997 considerable funding was devoted to create new intensive care units (ICUs) in leading hospitals. Continuing resource limitations made these new ICUs function more like regular hospital wards; the regular wards in turn often provide little more than care that should be available at a nursing home.

Remarkably, the health system has focused its decreased resources so efficiently that maternal and child mortality rates, already among the low-

---

[20] Rojas Ochoa and López Pardo (1997).

est in Latin America, continued to decline. Only among those over 65 did mortality rise (by ten per cent).[21] Besides the deterioration of hospital services, most of the 'costs' of the special period have been paid by the doctors. Deterioration in medical incomes has reduced the effective purchasing power of a physician's salary to about US$20 per month. This mattered little in the 1960s when the ration provided most basic goods and rent, transportation and electricity were essentially free. But with the deterioration of the ration basket of goods and increasing charges for basic services, the standard of living for Cuba's enormous pool of doctors is approaching misery. Distressing scenes of doctors moonlighting as prostitutes, taxi drivers or selling food to patients during rounds are expressions of this situation. Furthermore, MINSAP is unable to offer much in the way of professional incentives to doctors such as continuing education programmes, participation in international meetings or technical equipment. Deteriorating hospitals and impoverished physicians present the greatest limitations to the health system in the special period.

Universal access and state finance for all health services can only continue if all doctors are publicly employed. Indeed, while nurses and others are now permitted to operate small businesses or work in the tourist sector, physicians by law cannot. Cuba will face problems of health sector financing for an extended period; even if the economy grows at five per cent a year it will take 15 years for the national product to return to the level prior to the special period. At that time it will still not have access to funds like those that were available via subsidies from the Soviet Union which facilitated the growth of cradle-to-grave benefits. As an expression of success of previous social investments, the population above 65 has begun to expand rapidly and the social security system is already in financial crisis. The frail elderly will make increasing demands on the health system in the years ahead. Further reforms in the health system are needed to promote cost savings and regain efficiency in order to preserve its financial viability and resolve the grave problems that doctors and hospitals face.

Conclusions

Medicine has been a growing field in Cuba ever since half of the physicians left the country in the early 1960s.[22] For the first time since the Cuban revolution, unemployment among physicians is likely to occur. The government has responded with remarkable flexibility and ingenuity to preserve the regime to date. 'We are creating a new equilibrium based on a changed economic situation of our country. It is not the equilibrium of a developed country or of a poor country in a market economy. It is a model which is unknown; we have to create it as we go along.'[23]

---

[21] Garfield and Santana (1997).
[22] See Danielson (1979).
[23] Personal communication, Enrique Comandero, 18 Aug. 1997.

Efforts to maintain a one-class system of public medical care will founder unless productivity rises rapidly, restoring the value of *peso* salaries relative to the dollar. Today a taxi driver may earn fifty times more than a physician. Alternatively, 'escape valves' must be established to permit doctors to take part in the new private sector of the economy. This might result in the re-emergence of physicians as a privileged social group and would surely result in a health system with less social equity. Health leaders are determined to avoid this; dollarisation of the economy has already led to a two-class system of care. Private practice could eventually lead to the impoverishment of the public system of care, leaving it in the status as a charity system for indigents.

With the highest doctor-to-population ratios in the world and what might be the lowest medical income standards, changes are clearly ahead for Cuba. The challenge of preserving the programmes and systems associated with the lowest infant and maternal mortality rates in the developing world, in the context of economic decline and a privatising economy, will be instructive to the many other developing countries influenced by Cuban innovations since the 1960s.

CHAPTER 7

Health Reform and Policies for the Poor in Mexico

Octavio Gómez-Dantés

Reforms labelled as stabilisation and structural adjustment have been implemented across Latin America since the 1980s, and they have become associated with a disturbing increase in poverty and inequity in the region. According to the United Nations Economic Commission for Latin America and the Caribbean, between 1980 and 1990, the number of poor people in the region increased from 136 million to 196 million and the incidence of poverty rose from 41 to 46 per cent of the population.[1] Regarding inequity, Lustig states that income concentration in Latin America was also exacerbated in the 1980s, with the richest 20 per cent of the population earning incomes ten times greater than those of the poorest 20 per cent, which represented the worst income distribution of all the regions of the world.[2]

In order to address the most important adverse effects of the crisis and the process of adjustment on social wellbeing, most Latin American countries developed in the 1990s, with the support of international agencies, programmes for poverty alleviation and long-term investment in human capital. These mainly involved education and health services. The implementation of these programmes and investments reflected the recognition of two facts: that structural adjustment was taking longer to affect economic growth and poverty rates than many of its proponents originally believed; and that the delay could eventually influence the long-term sustainability of the economic reforms.[3]

In Mexico in the 1990s the Ministry of Health (MH) implemented two programmes — mostly financed with loans from the World Bank — directed to meet the basic health needs of the poorest sectors of the non-insured population. The first one, implemented between 1991 and 1995, was devoted to strengthening the physical infrastructure of the health services of the MH in the four poorest states of the country. The second one, the Programme for the Extension of Coverage (PEC), planned for the 1996–2000 period, intended to offer basic health services to the ten million Mexicans who had no regular access to healthcare in 1995.

In this chapter, the origins, initial results and prospects of this second programme will be discussed. First, a general overview of the health and healthcare situation in Mexico is presented, with a brief comment on the reform process of the Mexican healthcare system. Second, the challenges and prospects of the PEC are discussed. The main argument in this re-

---

[1] CEPAL (1993).
[2] Cited in Karl (1996).
[3] Zuvekas (1997).

gard is that in Mexico social programmes for the poor tend to constitute circumstantial responses to political pressures and, as such, have contributed very little to the development of what have been called *basic capabilities*. In the case of health in Mexico, strict monitoring of these programmes is required in order to guarantee access to all citizens living in poor areas to continuous, comprehensive and good quality healthcare.

Health needs

Mexico has a population of approximately 91 million, the second largest in Latin America. While 75 per cent of its inhabitants already live in urban areas, around 12 per cent still dwell in approximately 140,000 scattered and very small communities. According to the World Bank classification, Mexico is an 'upper middle-income country', with a gross domestic product (GDP) per capita in 1994 of US$2,780.[4] The country is currently undergoing a process of transition that touches all sectors of society. In demographic terms, its population is growing but the growth rate has decreased considerably in the last two decades; life expectancy is increasing and the elderly population is gaining importance. From the epidemiological point of view, Mexico is facing complex challenges. Common infections, though decreasing, have not been fully controlled, while chronic diseases and injuries already represent the main causes of death and disability (see Table 7.1). The country is also facing emerging problems — like AIDS and the health effects of environmental pollution — and re-emerging infections — malaria, dengue, tuberculosis and cholera — all of which compete for the scarce resources of the health system.

This so called *protracted transition* is coupled with a process that has been called *epidemiological polarisation*, an unequal distribution of health needs between the northern and southern states of the country, between urban and rural areas and among social classes.[5] For example, infant mortality is twice as high in the five poorest states than in the five richest states of the country. Adult mortality in the state of Oaxaca is comparable to that of India, while in the state of Nuevo León it is comparable to that of several European countries. The burden of disease is greater in rural areas (6.8 million DALYs)[6] than in urban centres (6.2 million DALYs), the difference being mostly due to premature death. Studies have found that children of women living in extreme poverty are 2.5 times more likely to die before the age of one than the children of women who are not poor.[7]

---

[4] Banco Interamericano de Desarrollo (BID, 1997).

[5] Frenk (1995).

[6] Disability-Adjusted Life Years. This is a standard measurement of the burden of ill health and premature death, favoured by organisations such as the World Bank.

[7] Frenk (1995).

Table 7.1: Main Causes of Death — Mexico 1997

N°	Causes	Number of deaths	Deaths per 100,000
1	Cardiovascular diseases	68,040	71.8
2	Cancer	51,254	54.1
3	Diabetes mellitus	36,027	38.0
4	Accidents	35,876	37.9
5	Cerebrovascular diseases	24,689	26.1
6	Chronic liver diseases	22,865	24.1
7	Pneumonia and influenza	19,867	21.0
8	Perinatal ailments	19,821	20.9
9	Violence	13,558	14.3
10	Nephritis and nephrosis	10,229	10.8
	Total deaths	**440,437**	**464.9**

Source: Dirección General de Estadística e Informática (1998).

The health system

The Mexican health system is made up of three basic components (see Figure 7.1). The first includes those governmental organisations providing services for the uninsured population, which amounts to approximately 50 per cent of the total population, mainly the rural and urban poor. The most important institution involved in the provision of services for this population is the MH. The second and largest component, the social security system — which provides services for around 40 per cent of the population — includes an institute covering workers in the formal private sector of the economy, the Mexican Institute for Social Security (IMSS), plus separate organisations for federal civil servants (ISSTE), some local government employees, the armed forces and the employees of the national oil company (PEMEX). The third component, the private sector, is made up of a collection of healthcare providers working in hospitals, ambulatory clinics, offices and folk medicine units on a for-profit basis. In theory, this component should provide services for around ten per cent of the Mexican population. However, according to the 1994 National Health Survey, 23 per cent of the people enrolled in social security agencies reported as their usual source of ambulatory care a private provider.[8] In the same vein, 46 per cent of those people with no social security benefits reported that their usual source of primary care was a private practitioner.

---

[8] Secretaría de Salud (1994).

Figure 7.1: Mexican Healthcare System

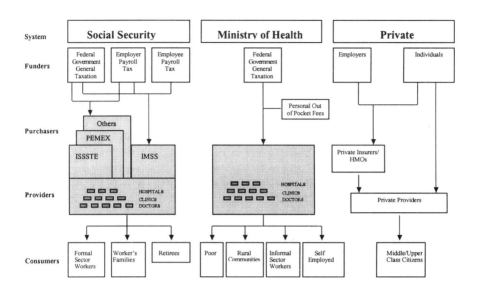

Health services for the poor are mainly organised through two channels. IMSS-Solidarity was established in 1979, to provide primary healthcare for the rural poor, and by 1995 was serving around 11 million people, according to official estimates. Although the institute is responsible for running this programme, it makes no direct financial contribution to it. Essentially, the IMSS contracts out its services to the federal government, but the services it provides have not been legally defined and the MH has no supervisory mandate. The primary healthcare needs of the urban poor are, in theory, provided for by the Ministry of Health.

Public institutions in Mexico are financed through three basic mechanisms. The agencies for the uninsured population are mainly financed with resources from the federal budget. Social security benefits for civil servants, the armed forces and other government-related groups are financed through employee contributions and a federal subsidy. Finally, the agency for private sector workers draws its resources from employees and employers' contributions and a federal subsidy. Regarding private expenditure, a large proportion of payments are made out of pocket and there is a small but growing voluntary medical insurance industry: five per cent of the urban population and two per cent of total health expenditure in 1994.[9]

Mexico spent 4.7 per cent of its GDP on healthcare in 1994 (see Table 7.2). Around half of the total resources were public (2.6 per cent) and half private (2.1 per cent). Per capita expenditure amounted to US$219. However, within public agencies this expenditure varied enormously, from more than US$400 per capita in PEMEX to US$19 in the MH.

---

[9] Knaul et al. (1997).

Table 7.2: Health Expenditure, Mexico 1992–96

Concept	Total Expenditure		Per Capita Expenditure		% GDP
	million pesos	dollars	million pesos	dollars	
Public Expenditure					
1992	28,560	9,211	329	106	2.6
1993	31,698	9,732	359	110	2.5
1994	37,320	10,946	415	122	2.6
1995/e	43,372	6,571	473	72	2.0
1996/e	53,081	6,894	569	74	2.4
Private Expenditure (low estimate)					
1992	30,697	9,901	354	114	2.7
1993	25,844	7,935	292	90	2.1
1994	29,952	8,785	333	98	2.1
1995/e	34,119	5,170	372	56	1.9
1996/e	43,648	5,669	468	61	2.0
Private Expenditure (high estimate)					
1992	30,697	9,901	354	114	2.7
1993	41,629	1,2781	471	145	3.3
1994	55,249	16,204	614	180	3.9
1995/e	ND	ND	ND	ND	ND
1996/e	ND	ND	ND	ND	ND
Total (low estimate)					
1992	49,843	16,076	574	185	4.5
1993	57,542	17,667	651	200	4.6
1994	67,272	19,730	747	219	4.7
1995/e	77,491	11,741	846	128	4.3
1996/e	96,729	12,562	1,038	135	4.4
Total (high estimate)					
1992	59,256	19,112	683	220	5.3
1993	73,324	22,513	829	255	5.8
1994	92,559	27,149	1,028	302	6.5
1995/e	ND	ND	ND	ND	ND
1996/e	ND	ND	ND	ND	ND

e – estimated figures

Source: Hernández et al. (1997).

The Mexican government, through the MH, has the responsibility for regulating the health system. However, there is little enforcement of regulations. The private sector, in particular, operates with very little outside monitoring. This is reflected in the poor quality of data available for this sector (see Table 7.2).

Key problems of the healthcare system

Since its inception in 1943, the modern Mexican healthcare system has consistently contributed to the reduction of mortality, the expansion of coverage, the provision of financial protection through the social security system, the training of human resources and the development of scientific research. However, the healthcare system is still facing several challenges, some of which will be discussed in this section.

Problems of access to healthcare

There are serious inequities in access to healthcare services. According to official figures, in 1995 ten per cent of the population had no regular access to basic healthcare services. If we also consider economic and organisational barriers, the number of Mexicans without regular access to basic health services could amount to at least 20 per cent of the national population.[10] A recent unpublished analysis of the 1994 National Health Survey found that of those who reported a serious health problem in the preceding 15 days but who did not seek attention, 51.8 per cent gave financial restrictions as the main cause.

Regarding access specifically to physicians, Mexico faces the contradiction of having medical urban unemployment but rural areas with no access to this kind of resource. In 1996, in the southern states of Chiapas, Hidalgo and Oaxaca there was one physician for every 1,108, 1,015 and 1,211 inhabitants, respectively: in contrast the northern state of Nuevo León had one physician for every 625 inhabitants.[11] Differences within states were even more extreme. In the state of Chiapas, the five municipalities with low levels of poverty had one physician for every 557 inhabitants, whereas the municipalities with an indigenous population in excess of 70 per cent had one physician for every 3,246 inhabitants.[12]

Shortages of beds and other inputs

Compared to all other upper middle-income countries of Latin America (Argentina, Brazil, Chile, Uruguay and Venezuela), Mexico has very few beds per unit of population (80.5/100,000).[13] The distribution of these beds is also highly uneven, with most facilities concentrated in urban areas, resulting in acute shortages in rural areas, especially the southern states of the country.

Basic inputs are also lacking. This is apparent in an unpublished MH evaluation of a programme to extend coverage to the poor implemented

---

[10] Frenk, González-Block and Lozano (1998).
[11] Dirección General de Estadística e Informática (1997).
[12] Frenk (1998a).
[13] Dirección General de Estadística e Informática (1997).

during the early 1990s (see below). The survey found that on average only 18 of the 36 drugs recognised to be essential for the most frequent health problems in poor areas were available. Basic antibiotics (ampicillin and penicillin), antimalarials and antituberculosis drugs were lacking in more than 50 per cent of the health centres surveyed.

Inefficiency

Overall, Mexico's spending patterns are inefficient. Health expenditure favours costly, non-communicable diseases in urban centres while little attention is given to primary interventions that could yield important savings to the system. In addition, less than ten per cent of public spending is devoted to preventive care, while curative services absorb almost 70 per cent. Inefficiencies are also manifest in the distribution of resources between administrative and medical activities. The social security agency for the state workers (ISSSTE), for example, devotes 33 per cent of its budget and 19 per cent of its personnel to administration. There are strong indications that the IMSS-Solidarity Programme has been suffering from particularly serious problems. Between 1988 and 1994 the number of rural health units under the programme grew by 47 per cent, but its population coverage only increased by an estimated three per cent. Likewise, the MH's efforts for the urban poor have been beset by extreme levels of bureaucratic fragmentation and no overall coordination.

Poor quality of care

Public sector agencies operate like a monopoly, hence, there is little consumer choice, few incentives for responsiveness to consumer needs and little concern for quality of care. In addition, many public sector hospitals are deteriorating in terms of infrastructure and supplies — probably due to the drastic cuts in public expenditures during the 1980s. Neither public nor private facilities are subject to regular processes of accreditation that verify their capacity to provide an acceptable standard of care and consequently quality of hospital services varies widely. One study revealed that a baby born in a MH hospital was three times more likely to die in its first seven days of life than a baby of the same weight born in an IMSS hospital. The researchers concluded that the difference was due largely to variations in the quality of care provided at the two facilities.[14] Another study, developed at the primary care units of the MH, reported that 73 per cent of consultations provided in these units displayed severe quality deficiencies.[15]

Health system reform

The present health administration is attempting to meet these challenges through the implementation of a health sector reform that includes changes in the social security system and changes in the MH. The general proposal is to reorganise the system by functions (provision, financing and regula-

[14] Bobadilla (1988).
[15] Durán (1990).

tion), rather than by population groups. In this new scenario the MH would eventually be responsible for coordinating, monitoring and regulating the system (including social security agencies and private sector institutions). The social security agencies and private insurers would be in charge of financing healthcare activities. Finally, a plurality of public and private providers would be responsible for the provision of personal health services.[16]

The most important specific changes in the social security system — legally based on a reform of the Social Security Law passed in December 1995 and initially implemented in July 1997 — are the following:

1. The 1995 Social Security Law transferred the administration of retirement and old age pensions from the IMSS to a new set of public and private entities known as Asociaciones de Fondos para el Retiro (AFOREs).[17] This has brought to an end the cross-subsidisation of the institute's health insurance schemes (which were in heavy deficit) by the large surpluses generated by its pension funds. In response to this, the federal government introduced a new financial scheme for the IMSS which increases the government subsidy to the healthcare component of this agency from four per cent of its annual budget to around 33 per cent and reduces the employers' and employees' contributions from 95 to 67 per cent. This expansion of government participation in social security financing will re-establish financial equilibrium in the IMSS but will impose a considerable burden on the federal budget. The government believes that these obligations could eventually be met with the resources generated by the implementation of additional incentives to formal sector employment and fewer incentives to tax evasion (see Figure 7.2). In the short run, however, there is concern about the possibility of meeting these financial obligations partly at the expense of resources for the non-insured population or resources for public health activities. The lack of political debate about a reform with such large distributional consequences is symptomatic of the lack of real representation of the non-insured groups in the Mexican political system.

2. The implementation of new regulations that will allow private firms to replace the services provided by the IMSS with private healthcare plans for their employees (*opt-out provision*). Although the details of this new policy remain under debate, it is likely that the Mexican government will stimulate competition among managed care organisations to contract with employers in order to provide the private sector workers with comprehensive health benefits. In addition to stimulating the insurance industry and the private delivery of healthcare, this provision is expected to reduce employment costs by eliminating double insuring, a common practice in many large firms. This initiative, however, may also stimulate

---

[16] This model conforms closely to that described by Frenk and Londoño in chapter 2 of this volume.

[17] Mesa-Lago (1997).

the exit from IMSS of those firms that mainly employ workers in the highest income levels and who very seldom use the services of this social security agency. Thus, the opting-out of the 'good risks' may leave the institution in a critical financial situation and with the responsibility for taking care of those who contribute less to the system but use it more. Previous experiences in Chile, Argentina and the Philippines show that for-profit insurance plans and managed care organisations are often able to avoid the enrolment of older people, the chronically ill and the disabled, in spite of the expensive efforts of the regulatory bodies.[18]

Figure 7.2: The New Premium Structure for the IMSS

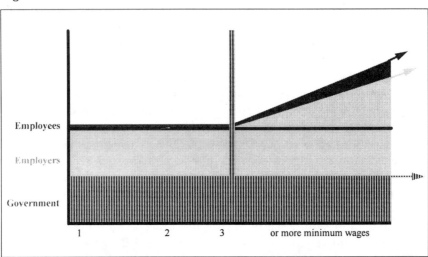

For all salaried workers, employers and the government will each contribute 13.9 per cent of the 1996 minimum wage (around US$14 per member per month), with the government contribution indexed to inflation and the employer's to the minimum salary in Mexico City. The share paid by employers will increase gradually to reach 20.4 per cent of the minimum wage by the year 2007. For workers earning more than three times the minimum wage, additional contributions will be paid as a fixed share of income: employers will pay six per cent of the wage above this level and employees will pay two per cent of the same portion. This total of eight per cent will be gradually reduced to 1.5 per cent over the next decade. By 2007, marginal rates of social security healthcare contribution on salaries above three times the minimum wage will be 0.4 per cent for workers and 1.1 per cent for employers, a change that is expected to reduce tax evasion. This final 1.5 per cent will be kept to meet a constitutional provision that demands a proportional element in social security contributions.

Source: Instituto Mexicano del Seguro Social (1997).

---

[18] Hsiao (1995); Stocker et al. (1999).

3. The creation of 131 newly decentralised Medical Area Units (MAUs), which include between one and three general hospitals and several clinics. Since January 1998 these have been receiving budget allocations based on a capitation formula adjusted for age and sex. These units are responsible for providing primary and secondary services to IMSS beneficiaries living in their catchment areas and will eventually be responsible for purchasing care for beneficiaries rather than providing it directly. These measures are intended to promote responsiveness to clients and local health needs and to stimulate efficiency.

4. The promotion of the affiliation of the members of the informal economy and the self-employed — mainly sectors of the urban population with the capacity to pay for better healthcare, but who do not belong to the formal economy — to the IMSS through a new plan financed with workers' contributions (in 1998 this contribution amounted to US$260 per year per nuclear family) and a subsidy from the federal government (around US$110) (Seguro de Salud para la Familia — *opt-in provision*). Four months after its inception, this new form of insurance had benefited 20,000 families and it is expected to extend to 350,000 families by the year 2000.[19] Nevertheless, this still only represents a small fraction of informal and self-employed workers. High levels of poverty among these occupation categories mean that the annual contribution is an insurmountable financial barrier for many, regardless of the health benefits.

5. It was proposed that all responsibility for IMSS-Solidarity's activities be transferred from the institute to the newly-decentralised state health authorities (see below). This policy was strongly resisted by the IMSS, although it was agreed that services would in future be contracted at the state rather than federal level. However, there are few signs of this happening as yet.

The reforms of the Ministry of Health include the following:

1. The completion of the decentralisation process of health services for the uninsured population that had been initiated in 1987. A gradual process is anticipated. State health services will first take up the functions of the MH and eventually will merge with other decentralised institutions that presently are taking care of important portions of the uninsured population, such as IMSS-Solidaridad. However, the challenge of this process, which has enormous potential in Mexico, is to implement it according to the development of managerial abilities at the local level. Previous experiences in Latin America have shown that a badly planned and implemented decentralisation process may extend rather than solve local health problems, including questions of inequity.

---

[19] Instituto Mexicano del Seguro Social (IMSS, 1998).

2. The delivery of a package of 12 interventions to the ten million Mexicans who until 1995 had no regular access to basic health services. The logic, initial results and perspectives of this initiative, known as the Programme for the Extension of Coverage (PEC), will be discussed in the section that follows.

3. The Programme of Education, Health and Nutrition for the Extreme Poor (PROGRESA) was implemented in 1997. It seeks to identify families in greatest need and to offer them cash incentives for participation in basic health and education activities. It involves collaboration between the MH and other state agencies at the federal and local levels. However, by late 1998 the programme had yet to become operational in most of the country.

4. Finally, in February 1998, the MH implemented a new and ambitious policy intended to increase the availability and regular prescription of generic drugs. A catalogue of 74 generic drugs was designed by the MH and these drugs are already being distributed by many drugstores all over the country at considerably lower prices than commercial pharmaceuticals. The intention is to gradually increase the number of drugs in the catalogue to eventually include all products of the list of essential drugs of public institutions.

Programme for the Extension of Coverage

Several healthcare programmes for the poor have been implemented in the last 30 years in Mexico: the Programme of Mobile Healthcare Units for Rural Areas (1971); the Rural Health Programme (1979); the Healthcare Programme for Marginalised Populations in Large Urban Areas (1981); and the Strategy for Extension of Coverage (1985). In the last decade, in the context of a structural adjustment, two additional programmes were developed: the Support Programme for Healthcare Services for the Non-Insured Population (PASSPA) (1991–95) and the PEC (1996-2000).

The main objective of PASSPA was to strengthen the healthcare infrastructure of the primary healthcare units of the MH in the four poorest states of the country (Chiapas, Guerrero, Hidalgo and Oaxaca). Through this programme, per capita healthcare expenditure gaps were reduced[20] and potential regular access to healthcare was extended to almost two million people. However, even though the MH implemented a thorough evaluation of the programme, little else is known about its real impact, since the results of this exercise were never disseminated. For example, there is no publicly available information about the utilisation rates of the units affected by the programme, the quality of care or the availability of essential drugs.

---

[20] Lara et al. (1997).

The PEC, on the other hand, intends to extend basic healthcare coverage to those 10 million Mexicans who lacked such services in 1995 through the supply of a package of services which includes the following 12 interventions:

1. Basic household sanitation measures

2. Family planning

3. Prenatal, natal and postnatal care

4. Nutrition and growth surveillance

5. Immunisation

6. Treatment of diarrhoea at the household level

7. Treatment of common parasitic diseases

8. Treatment of acute respiratory infections

9. Prevention and control of tuberculosis

10. Prevention and control of hypertension and diabetes

11. Prevention of accidents and initial treatment of injuries

12. Community training for health promotion

The programme and the package —designed through a normative exercise developed at the National Council of Health (a recently re-established forum headed by the national minister of health and comprising the ministers of health of the 32 states of the Mexican Federation) — were implemented in response to several considerations. The growing influence of utilitarian perspectives within the health sector all over the world has emphasised the implementation of cost-effective interventions, which in developing countries tend to target the rural poor. At the same time, international demands for 'adjustment with a human face' have spurred multilateral banks to revise their policies in order to protect vulnerable groups from the most adverse effects of economic reforms. Finally, the enormous national and international pressure generated by the revolt in the southern state of Chiapas in 1994 created additional reasons to implement and extend this programme.

The basic package is being offered in 18 states of the federation through a special programme financed with a loan from the World Bank and resources from the MH. Two basic schemes are being used in its implementation: geographical and functional extension. Geographical extension is directed to the most dispersed communities with no healthcare facilities, and it implies the supply of these interventions through mobile medical teams and primary healthcare workers, mostly recruited from the target communities. Functional extension means strengthening the physical, human and organisational infrastructure of the existing rural facilities. According to official figures, two years after its inception, the PEC had reached 18 states, 600 municipalities and six million people.[21]

Prospects of the PEC and healthcare for the poor

The effort implied in the PEC in terms of the mobilisation of financial, managerial, human and technical resources is enormous. The problems that this programme is trying to address are probably the most challenging of all those presently confronted by the MH. In organisational terms there is nothing as difficult, demanding and potentially more frustrating as a programme for the extension of coverage for dispersed populations in a context of limited resources. Without any disregard for the efforts implied in such an endeavour, some of its limitations and its prospects will be discussed.

The fundamental failing of the PEC is that the problems it is trying to solve are being presented in such a way as to limit the government's responsibility for the prevailing inequities which underpin them. This is hardly surprising, given that the same political party governed Mexico from the beginning of the century until its eventual defeat in July 2000. Partly because of this, the PEC avoids a serious commitment to the solution to these problems. The general figures on coverage presented to the public by the government officials in charge of the PEC underestimate the seriousness of unmet basic needs which require a large injection of additional resources and, above all, structural changes to the healthcare system. Without a detailed picture of the health problems this programme is supposed to confront; without a serious discussion regarding the possible causes of these problems; and without close monitoring of the implementation of the PEC, it will be difficult to call public health officials to account and to guarantee the fulfilment of the goals of the programme.

As Frenk has stated, persistent inequity is the most characteristic feature of the health status of Mexico.[22] However, this fact has not been sufficiently stressed in official circles, probably due to the fact that resource allocation policies within the health sector have contributed to such a situation. Public expenditure on health has traditionally favoured the insured population and, within the MH, the capital city and the northern states, the least needy regions of the country. Thus, when health expenditure per capita is disaggregated by public institution, twentyfold differences are detected. Likewise, per capita expenditure for the non-insured population in the northern region is double that of

---

[21] Secretaría de Salud (1997).
[22] Frenk (1998b).

central states and treble that of southern ones.[23] These figures, on the one hand, suggest that the strategic importance and the negotiating abilities of the states determine resource allocation in the health sector in Mexico. On the other hand, these figures contradict the main principle implied in the concentration of an important amount of taxes in the federal realm: its redistribution from the most developed areas to the most needy ones. It was in response to this situation that the MH designed a new resource allocation formula using indicators such as the marginality index and infant mortality rate. However, this formula is being used only to allocate fresh resources, a fact that will limit its potential impact.

Another concern is that the government may limit its commitment to the poor to offering the package of 12 interventions, which is by any standards a very limited offer. This may leave the inequity within the system untouched, especially if the government does not address at the same time the fact that the better off have access to a much wider range of services subsidised by the public purse.[24] In fact, the recent increase of the government financing of the main social security agency may serve to worsen such inequities.

In general terms, however, nobody in the country opposes the PEC, mainly because it is not affecting the present distribution of resources (since it is mostly financed by a foreign loan), nor does it damage any of the important interest groups in the health sector: physicians, the pharmaceutical industry, unions and private providers. However, there are no local advocacy groups or political parties specifically following it or demanding its reasonable implementation, as opposed, for example, to the reform of the social security agencies. Even though it is directed at a population of at least ten million people, this population tends to attract limited attention, due to its dispersity and lack of organisation, its considerable physical distance from the national capital — and even from the state capitals — and its low voter turnout.[25]

This explains why the MH can announce the extension of coverage to six million people in two years — a figure difficult to believe — without receiving almost any reaction from the press or the mass media. Only a year after this announcement, the Pan American Health Organisation stated that 'only seven Mexican states had demonstrated full health services coverage'.[26]

And even if these six million people are now receiving some sort of healthcare, in the short run there are many more things that the public needs to know. We need to know whether these people are really part of the target populations and whether or not they are using the available services. We need information on the number of interventions they now have access to and whether they have access to these interventions on a regular basis or through mobile teams visiting the communities at long intervals. We also need information on the technical and interpersonal quality of the care they are receiving and on the availability of basic healthcare inputs — most notably, essential drugs.

---

[23] Lara et al. (1997).
[24] Mills (1998).
[25] Reich (1995).
[26] Cruz (1999).

Conclusion

Major changes will be needed to guarantee consistent access of the rural, dispersed populations of Mexico to comprehensive healthcare. First of all, additional resources for the social sector would have to be negotiated with the central and state governments. Within the health sector, the inequities of the traditional distribution of public resources between social security agencies and the agencies for the non-insured population will have to be confronted. The recent increase of the federal government's participation in financing social security agencies may create problems by widening expenditure gaps among public institutions. Finally, within the MH, resource allocation patterns among states and between different levels of care will have to be modified. All of these structural changes, however, would generate distributional and political consequences that demand enormous will and ability from those groups within and outside the MH who are seeking to improve the access to healthcare for the worse-off.

In the short run, a close follow-up of the process of implementation of healthcare programmes for the poor will be needed. Working alone, the health authorities will do little to promote this, due to their lack of a monitoring and evaluation culture and the absence of formal accountability mechanisms in the country. Political groups, NGOs and academic centres could help fill the voids in this respect.

Berlin used to state that the first public obligation is to avoid the extremes of suffering.[27] For this single reason, programmes directed to meet the basic health needs of the poor are justified. However, in the long run, these programmes should avoid becoming survival interventions and turn into programmes for the development of health understood as a *basic capability*. This capability does not mean being healthy all the time, but having access to the means of prevention of all sorts of diseases and, in case of disease, to a comprehensive system of healthcare capable of reducing to a minimum the loss of productivity related to these events.[28]

In the development of health policies for the poor in Mexico, proposals for the integration of the services for the poor with those of more powerful groups should be considered. Public health professionals know very well that services for the poor tend to be poor services. To move away from such a discouraging tradition in the design of health programmes, the needs of the poor will have to be met through services that also attend the healthcare demands of more vocal and organised sectors of society.

---

[27] Berlin (1992).
[28] Trejo and Jones (1993).

CHAPTER 8

Healthcare Financing, Reform and Equity in Argentina: Past and Present

Peter Lloyd-Sherlock

Many Latin American countries have recently begun to implement sweeping health sector reforms. These policies have sought to respond to a variety of challenges, including demographic, epidemiological and technological changes, as well as a major redefinition of the role of the public sector.[1] Argentina is no exception to this regional trend, and from the early 1990s its healthcare system was receiving increased attention from politicians, policy-makers and international agencies such as the World Bank, United Nations Development Programme (UNDP) and the Inter-American Development Bank (IADB). These saw existing arrangements as inefficient and out of step with the new social, economic and welfare structures that the Menem administrations had been in the process of imposing. A series of reforms were proposed, most of which are now being implemented. Already, the Argentine experience is being vaunted as a resounding success and another essential step in the modernisation of its economic and social structures. The IADB recently described the changes as: '... the greatest transformation of a healthcare system in Latin America during the 1990s'.[2] Rather than redefine policy goals, the change of government in January 2000 has led to a deepening of the Menemist project.

The Argentine reforms can be divided into two largely separate areas. First, there have been attempts to replace the rigid monopoly of the union-run *obra social* occupational insurance funds with more flexible, consumer-led private provision. This has essentially entailed a merger of the social insurance with the private insurance sectors, both of which are theoretically to operate within a new regulatory framework. Secondly, there have been a range of reforms in the publicly financed healthcare sector, including decentralisation, the establishment of hospital trusts and the conversion of specialist doctors into general practitioners. The former set of reforms seeks to promote the role of the free market in healthcare financing. The latter set is concerned with developing an effective safety net for market failures and to refocus public sector attention towards primary healthcare.

It is essential that Argentina's reforms be put into a historical perspective, both in order to understand the nature of the problems and structures being changed and to learn from earlier reform experiences. Such a review must go back at least as far as the early twentieth century, since it will become apparent that the health systems of that period already contained

---

[1] See Londoño and Frenk in this volume.
[2] Inter-American Development Bank (1998).

similar characteristics and problems to the present day. Key long-standing weaknesses include an inappropriate segmentation of financing and provision, ineffectual regulation and an overall lack of equity in terms of both financing and health outcomes. The review shows that healthcare reform had been repeatedly attempted throughout the century, but that many proposals were either never legislated for or were ineffectually implemented. This raises doubts about the feasibility of the current project. If, notwithstanding these doubts, the Menem reforms and those of the new administration are judged a success, it is necessary to establish what may have changed to allow this to happen and whether the reforms will resolve underlying problems of equity and institutional weakness.

Healthcare before the 1940s

Studies of Argentina's healthcare system are available from the late nineteenth century. These show a level of infrastructural development comparable to that of Australia and Canada.[3] However, they also reveal a high degree of segmentation in both financing and provision. Health insurance funds were already well developed in Buenos Aires and the larger industrial centres, operating through two types of organisation. By 1914, over 200 mutual aid societies provided for around 300,000 affiliates in the capital city alone (19 per cent of its total population).[4] Nevertheless, large sections of the population remained unprotected by these schemes. Most mutual aid societies were run by labour organisations and primarily catered for working men. Indeed, women were often expressly barred from joining and before the 1940s most societies did not extend cover to direct dependants. Partly because of this, the range of services offered was relatively limited. There was little provision for mother and child health and costly, long-term care was usually left to the public hospitals. Moreover, few societies actually owned medical facilities, but instead contracted out to third party providers. Also, the fixed capitation system of payments favoured by most societies led to a fairly minimalistic approach to service provision.[5]

While mutual aid societies made a significant contribution to the health and welfare of a large section of the population, they suffered from numerous important problems. Societies were extremely varied in terms of size and the services they offered. In 1927 the six largest societies accounted for 60 per cent of total affiliation, whereas 55 societies accounted for only five per cent. Levels of efficiency also varied considerably, with little apparent relationship between contribution rates and the extent or quality of services. The fragmented and piecemeal nature of the mutual aid sector was of particular concern since government supervision of the societies was virtually non-existent.[6]

---

[3] Veronelli (1975); Recalde (1991).

[4] Rough calculation made by Bunge (1917).

[5] For a good summary of different payment methods in health insurance and their effect on service quality, see Mills (1983).

[6] In 1914 a reform bill was unsuccessfully proposed, which would have created a supervisory agency, imposed a minimum size of 200 affiliates, stipulated that at least 80 per cent of contri-

Mutual aid societies showed little interest in poorer sections of the workforce, whose only alternative was to join disreputable 'health firms' (*empresas sanitarias*). These health firms had a membership of around 90,000 in Buenos Aires in 1914. They levied smaller contributions than the mutual aid societies and provided a markedly inferior service. Indeed, numerous official reports characterised them as parasitic and of no real benefit to the welfare of workers. According to one medical journal of the day:

> A doctor without conscience and an unscrupulous businessman team up to get rich at the expense of sick paupers. The businessman does the rounds of the tenements and poor houses, seeking out affiliates for the newly formed firm. He promises the world: doctors, medicines, pensions, funeral expenses, a trip to Europe, etc., etc. All this for the modest sum of one and a half *pesos* a month. The doctor is responsible for the other side of the farce. He calls on the sick in such a hurry that he never discovers what illness they actually have and makes out prescriptions which are so cheap that in no case will they exceed 50 *centavos*. When there is a very serious illness, a caesarean section or the like, the patient is immediately bundled off to the Assistance Hospital.[7]

Thus even before the First World War, health insurance in Argentina was highly stratified and fragmented. Mutual aid societies catered for the more privileged sections of the workforce; health firms covered relatively less affluent groups while the remainder of the population, typically those engaged in rural activities outside Buenos Aires, had no health insurance cover of any kind.

Hospital facilities displayed a similar pattern of fragmentation. A survey of Buenos Aires conducted in 1887 found hospitals administered by the federal and municipal government, as well as the private sector, which included both profit and non-profit making organisations.[8] Little coordination occurred between the different types of hospital and it was claimed that public ones suffered from serious overcrowding, whereas private ones generally enjoyed superior facilities and excess capacity.[9] Per capita expenditure also varied sharply with far lower levels in the

---

butions should be used solely for health services and laid down a framework for public hospitals to contract out services to the societies. Only in 1932 was a minimal level of state regulation imposed (Katz and Muñoz, 1988, pp.73–9)

[7] *La Mutualidad*, vol. 3, no. 8, p. 5 (1905), cited in Katz and Muñoz (1988). Similar criticisms were made by Buenos Aires Council and the Department of National Hygiene.

[8] There were two sorts of non-profit hospitals. A small number of large facilities were constructed by immigrants of specific nations to provide services mainly for their own national communities. These included the Italian Hospital (founded in 1826) and the British Hospital (1844). Secondly, there were hospitals run by 'philanthropic societies'. The term 'philanthropic' should not be equated with charitable, since most of the beneficiaries were from relatively privileged sections of society, rather than the poor. For a detailed account of hospital facilities in this period, see Recalde (1991). Virtually no information is available about the for-profit sector (a problem which is also apparent in the present day).

[9] Various efforts were made to centralise hospital administration but none were successful. A detailed account of these initiatives is available in Veronelli (1975), pp. 51–62.

public sector. Mutual aid societies had developed contractual arrangements with the private sector rather than public hospitals, which were seen as worse than second rate. As such, there was a clear division of public provision for the poor and private provision for the privileged.

Cross subsidisation between the public and private sectors was also a key feature of this period. As well as overlaps of personnel and utilisation, there were direct transfers from the public purse to private operators. No precise figures are available, but reports from the period observe that government transfers accounted for an increasingly significant proportion of mutual aid society revenue.[10] These funds were not allocated on a systematic basis and it is claimed that more often than not they targeted the richer and more powerful societies.[11] Similarly, the non-profit making hospitals received substantial donations from all levels of government. In 1904 the largest philanthropical society, the Sociedad de Beneficencia, alone received 50 per cent more funding than that allocated to all the country's public hospitals put together.[12]

The data do not allow for a full empirical survey of the distributional effect of healthcare financing, but the above account leaves little room for doubt about the system's strong overall regressive impact, both in terms of financing and health. The healthcare system also displayed a sharp geographical bias, with services and facilities highly concentrated in the richest cities and regions. The segmented and fragmented structure of healthcare reflected a complex interplay of political pressures rather than economic realities and social needs. More powerful and economically privileged groups enjoyed superior healthcare services, which attracted disproportionate levels of financing. Even within the mutual aid societies, privileged groups were able to obtain exclusive status. In some cases, for example, executives would be entitled to join a separate society from the rest of the workforce employed by the same firm. The result was a highly complex and inefficient structure, whose guiding principle was social exclusivity rather than solidarity. If the Argentine healthcare system was remarkably well developed by the early twentieth century, then so were its structural weaknesses. Interestingly, many of these were very similar to problems identified in the 1990s, as will be seen below.

Competing models (1940s and '50s)

1944 saw a major political watershed in Argentine history with the installation of the first Peronist administration. The early years of Peronist governance were strongly inclined towards the union sector (which was its major source of political support) and to a more egalitarian social model. They also advocated

---

[10] Garuffi (1939), cited in Katz and Muñoz (1988).
[11] For example, in 1936 the Senate approved a 300,000 *peso* grant to the powerful railway workers' fund (Belmartino et al., 1991, p. 104).
[12] Katz and Muñoz (1988), p. 102.

the imposition of a corporatist, state-led model of development along similar lines to those pursued by fascist governments in southern Europe.

With regard to health policy, there was a clear contradiction in the overall Peronist ideology. By this period, the great majority of mutual aid societies were administered by trade unions.[13] Indeed, they provided the unions with their principal sources of financing and, arguably, of their political power. As such, the unions sought the strengthening of an autonomous mutual aid society sector, which would remain structured along occupational divisions. This vision was clearly at odds with the government's strong commitment to a universal, uniform and egalitarian state-led welfare model. It was this contradiction which gave rise to the sharp divide between the insurance and non-insurance health sectors, which has remained a major feature of the healthcare system ever since.

The new government's statist orientation was reflected in its desire to bring the mutual aid societies under much stronger central control than had hitherto been the case. In 1946 all mutual aid societies were brought directly under the control of the powerful Labour and Welfare Secretariat.[14] This did not, however, see any reduction in the dominant role played by the unions. First, the Secretariat was itself largely run by union leaders at this time. Second, the regulation of mutual aid societies remained extremely lax and they therefore retained a very large measure of operational autonomy. Nevertheless, the change in the nominal status of the mutual aid sector was heralded as a major step towards an embracing state welfare system. The reform was formalised with the gradual remodelling of mutual aid societies into so-called 'social works agencies' or *obras sociales*: a measure which was largely cosmetic and which distracts from the essential continuity of health insurance provision over this period.[15] The only significant developments were a surge in overall affiliation, due to the growth of trade union membership and an increased tendency for funds to provide services directly (although the bulk were still contracted out).[16] Far greater change was seen in the public healthcare sector. In 1946 the status of the government agency responsible for this area was upgraded to secretariat level and placed under the leadership of Ramón Carrillo, an influential Peronist figure. This was followed by an unprecedented expansion of public hospitals and the adoption of major public health campaigns to eradicate such illnesses as malaria. Between 1946 and 1951 the total number of hospital beds in Argentina increased from 66,300 to 114,609, with

---

[13] For an account of the shift of mutual aid societies away from ethnic groups to a union structure, see Munck (1998).

[14] Mensa (1946).

[15] The first *obra social* (for railway workers) was established in 1944 and by 1955 virtually all the old mutual aid societies had been 'transformed'. Both types of organisation were essentially autonomous and unregulated. Both were mainly administered by unions and contracted out the majority of health services. *Obras sociales* remained extremely heterogeneous and fragmented both in terms of size and services.

[16] Not all occupation groups were granted *obras sociales*. For example, several proposals to develop funds for sugar workers were ignored. This group was poorly organised, with few links with the national Peronist power structure (Belmartino et al., 1991, pp. 126–7).

almost all of the increase accounted for by the public sector. Efforts were made to promote hospital construction in under-served parts of the interior in order to compensate for pre-existing geographical inequalities of health provision. This expansion was a major step towards developing an effective universal public healthcare system. At the same time, government funding for the non-profit hospitals was discontinued and most of them were incorporated into either the public or the for-profit sectors.

As such, the 1940s and '50s saw the consolidation of two quite contradictory rival healthcare models. Even by the early 1950s, the Public Health Secretariat still saw the participation of the mutual aid societies and *obras sociales* as merely a transitional step towards the development of a universal national health service. Conversely, the Secretariat of Labour and Welfare was loath to surrender responsibility for health insurance and had a very different vision of the future. According to Katz and Muñoz:

> The fact that medical social insurance developed through the *obra social* system and in association with the trade unions ... gave rise to the emergence of a profound legal conflict which has continued up to the present day ... between the Ministry of Health and the Labour and Welfare Ministry ... which has meant that health has been systematically treated as an element of political negotiation between the state and the unions and not as an end in itself.[17]

These institutional divisions and conflicts have remained the dominant characteristic of Argentine healthcare until the 1990s. While the general expansion of healthcare was a major achievement, the failure to adopt a global model was to have a more lasting impact.

The emergence of the contemporary healthcare system (1960s to '90s)

After the military overthrow of Perón in 1955, various proposals were made to substantially reform the *obras sociales*. There was much criticism about continued inequities, poor service quality and crushing bureaucracy throughout the insurance sector. However, reform proposals had to take account of a range of interest groups, which had attained increased significance by this time. Although this period was characterised more by military dictatorship than democratic civilian rule, the expansion of the modern urban labour force afforded trade unions continued political influence. Furthermore, bodies specifically representing medical interests, such as the Confederación Médica de la República Argentina (COMRA — Argentine Federation of Doctors), enjoyed unprecedented power and influence.

A combination of frequent regime changes and the resistance of interest groups delayed the passage of any substantial reform until the late 1960s. The main reform bill, enacted in 1970, established the structure of health insurance that has survived up to the present day. Among the more important aspects of the bill were the imposition of obligatory affiliation for all

---

[17] Katz and Muñoz (1988), pp. 35–6.

sectors of the workforce and the creation of a new supervisory body, the Instituto Nacional de Obras Sociales (INOS). The Institute was to ensure that the health services provided through *obras sociales* complied with minimum government standards, was empowered to audit the *obras* and to establish a Fondo de Redistribución (FDR). This fund was designed to compensate for inequities within the health insurance sector by redistributing income from richer *obras sociales* to less affluent ones.[18] Further legislation sought, for the first time, to regulate the nature of contracts between insurers and providers. If they had been fully implemented in the way intended by the bill, these reforms would have gone a long way to increase the efficiency and equity of the health insurance sector. It will, however, become apparent that this was far from the case.

The spectacular expansion of the public hospital infrastructure witnessed during the previous period was not sustained. Indeed, between 1958 and 1980 the number of hospital beds provided by this sector actually fell (from 97,319 to 94,883). The trend was in stark contrast to the boom in private provision (mainly contracting to the *obras*), where hospital beds increased from 17,903 to 47,048 over the same period. Within the public health budget there were substantial cuts in overall funding, along with attempts to promote the decentralisation of overall administrative and financial responsibility to provincial governments and to encourage the adoption of user fees.[19] None of this was done systematically. Plans for decentralisation were essentially spurred by the short-term financial difficulties of the federal government, rather than by any desire to promote flexibility, accountability or participation. Implementation was often inconsistent and confused. A more systematic decentralisation was not begun until the early 1980s. Similarly, the implementation of user fees was unregulated and ineffective and very little progress was made in recouping from the *obras* the costs of treating insurance affiliates. The provision of insufficient funds for hospital maintenance caused a marked deterioration in equipment and buildings. As such, the gap between the quality of service provided by the private sector and the public one (with the exception of a small number of prestigious high-tech hospitals) widened considerably.

The 1980s saw the emergence of a significant private health insurance sector for the first time since 1945. Between 1974 and 1989 the number of private insurers grew from 25 to over 200. This sector was entirely unregulated and many insurers functioned primarily as financial organisations, taking advantage of spiralling inflation rates. To this end, many private firms followed the abusive traditions of the old *empresas sanitarias*. According to a later report:

---

[18] *Obras sociales* were obliged to contribute ten per cent of their income from affiliates' contributions and 60 per cent of any other income to the FDR.

[19] These processes gathered intensity during the 1980s. For example, between 1980 and 1986 per capita spending on public health fell from 28.2 to 12.1 1980 US dollars.

Since the private health sector was unregulated, any charlatan could set up shop. With no minimum requirements for assets or liquidity limiting market entry, consumers were unprotected from those that chose to defraud members. The *prepagas* [private insurers] often introduced all kinds of exclusion clauses into their contracts. Plans and premiums were frequently changed without customers being notified.[20]

Rather than direct state intervention, it was the virtual elimination of inflation from 1991 that brought about the end of such abusive practices. The number of private insurers fell sharply and the market consolidated, with rapid concentration into a small number of large firms.

Taking the healthcare system as a whole, the 1950s, '60s and '70s saw the triumph of the occupation-specific *obra social* model over the unified, non-contributory one. This occurred despite the best efforts of several governments to develop a single national health service, incorporating both sectors. The first attempt to do so, led by a newly installed Peronist government in the early 1970s, failed in the face of concerted resistance from a range of actors. According to Belmartino and Bloch:

> The strong opposition of the unions determined that the project for the incorporation of the *obras sociales* [into the national health service] was of a voluntary nature, which meant in practice that it never happened ... The project affected very powerful interests and very strongly held views about the healthcare system. Private medical providers, the pharmaceutical industry and even health professionals were convinced of the merits of a flexible system ... But the weight of trade union opposition must have been at least as important as all the rest combined, taking into account that this constituted one of the principal tenets of the national power structure [of the pro-union Peronist government].[21]

By contrast, the violently repressive military regime that followed (1976–83) was able virtually to eliminate the trade unions as political actors. Control of the *obras sociales* was taken away from the unions and given to individuals nominated by the de facto national president. In this context, it might have been expected that more effective policies could have been imposed. Very little was achieved, however. In this case, the continued resistance of pharmaceutical companies and professional bodies, such as COMRA, to change was as effective as the unions had been before. Finally, a more concerted reform effort was made in the mid-1980s by the democratic Alfonsín administration. Once again, the resistance of strong vested interests (in this case, an alliance between the Peronists, then in opposition, and traditional unions) was able to block legislation.[22]

Meanwhile, it was apparent that the regulatory system developed in the 1970 bill was far from effective. Even officials of the military government admitted that:

[20] Justo (1998), p. 64.
[21] Belmartino and Bloch (1982).
[22] Belmartino and Bloch (1994).

The open failure of the INOS and the consequent lack of effective controls
has brought about numerous irregularities, such as the partial or total disappearance of contributions, the failure to provide adequate cover to important
sectors of beneficiaries and the diversion of the *obra sociales'* income towards
the financing of activities in which they should not be engaged.[23]

Numerous new bills sought to give INOS real teeth and to reduce political
interference and corruption in its functioning, which had reached crisis
proportions. However, following redemocratisation and the return of *obra*
management to the trade unions, it was clear that the system remained as
ineffectual as ever. A major World Bank study of the country's healthcare
system carried out in 1987 was particularly critical of the Redistribution
Fund.[24] First, it noted that the *obras* would often delay payment to the fund,
so that contributions were devalued by inflation. More importantly, the
fund's income was not transferred to those *obra sociales* providing lower
grade services to poorer populations (as was originally envisaged). Instead,
income was channelled to whichever *obra* had an end of year financial deficit: in practice, this usually meant those funds which offered better quality
services to richer groups. Consequently, rather than rewarding economic
efficiency or promoting progressive redistribution, the fund operated according to a principle of 'reverse solidarity' (the World Bank's own expression). Another World Bank survey conducted in 1996 found that, despite its
previous recommendations and the efforts of the Argentine government,
the insurance sector continued to suffer from similar problems. As regards
the Redistribution Fund, it observed that 'equity criteria were frequently
overruled in practice by political considerations ...' and added that '... *obras*
have not been required to obtain independent financial audits and only a
few have actually submitted data [to the official regulator] on their members, benefits structure and contracts'.[25]

These repeated failures to implement reform call into question the real
political will of successive governments to follow through in the face of
concerted opposition from a range of often powerful interest groups. Lack
of will was strongly conditioned by the low priority generally afforded
these issues in the national political agenda. Powerful actors such as the
unions and the pharmaceutical industry opposed measures that might
diminish their influence and autonomy. Under Peronist rule, the interests
of the unions were almost identical to those of the Labour Ministry, in
which the INOS was based. Even at other times there was at the very least
a strong 'sympathy' (if not an outright alliance) between the ministry's desire to maintain the status quo (namely a health system mainly organised
along the lines of occupational insurance) and the goals of the pharmaceutical companies, private clinics and (save during repressive regimes)
the unions. The Ministry of Labour and unions were interested in placing

---

[23] Taken from the text of Law 2,269 (1980), cited in Katz and Muñoz (1988), p. 51.
[24] World Bank (1987).
[25] World Bank (1997), pp. 12–13 and 19.

other concerns, such as collective bargaining, social pacts and labour legislation on the national agenda, while clinics and companies preferred to avoid the political limelight altogether. Symbolic politics also served to keep health insurance reform off the agenda. One clear example of this was the use of language by the media to exclude or label as marginal non-insured sections of the population.[26] This was associated with a marked lack of academic interest in health reform, as is made evident by the lack of published studies before the late 1980s. The combination of these effects and the perceived difficulty of implementation served to discourage politicians from raising the profile of the failed process.

Despite failures to reform the *obras sociales*, the imposition of obligatory affiliation in 1970 led to a major expansion of insurance coverage over the following decade (see Table 8.1). Expansion continued after 1979, although it was concentrated in those *obras* managed by provincial governments. Rather than resulting from a planned decentralisation policy, this reflected changes in the labour market. During the 1980s, the impact of a contracting private sector formal economy was largely offset by employment generation within provincial government bureaucracies. Much of this provincial employment was of minimal productivity and has been widely characterised as an anti-unemployment safety net.[27]

Table 8.1: Membership of *obras sociales*, 1967/8 to 1995

	National and provincial *obras*	Provincial *obras*	Military and police *obras*
1967/8	7,085,800	1,220,700	no data
1979	18,537,900	3,300,000	700,000
1990	18,800,000	no data	no data
1994	16,401,000	no data	no data
1995	16,271,000	no data	no data

Sources: González García et al. (1987), p. 52; World Bank (1993), p. 75; INDEC (1996), p. 316.

[26] A clear case of this was when a left-wing newspaper published a survey in 1992, which claimed that half of Argentines with unsatisfied basic needs were elderly people with insurance pensions, but made no reference to the roughly 25% of over 65 year-olds lacking both pension and health insurance (*Página 12*, 25 Nov. 1992).
[27] World Bank (1993b).

Some doubts have been voiced about the reliability of official affiliation statistics. For example, according to some official reports, 74.6 per cent of the total population had access to some form of *obra social*,[28] yet the 1991 official national census figure put it at only 58 per cent. Since 1993, the reduction of private formal sector employment has been dramatic and there have been concerted efforts to 'downsize' the bloated provincial bureaucracies. It is to be expected, then, that overall affiliation to *obras sociales* at both the national and provincial level will have fallen quite sharply from the mid-1990s. As such, the period up to the 1980s can be characterised as a time of steady expansion of health insurance, the 1980s as 'artificial expansion' (through unproductive provincial employment) and the 1990s as a time of stagnation and retrenchment. In this context, it is clear that the failure to develop a uniform, universal public health system was a major setback in the extension and completion of a rationally structured health system for the whole population.

A further problem was the pattern of resource allocation and service provision across the entire healthcare system. The failure to establish effective mechanisms to regulate contracts between *obras sociales* and private providers led to the emergence of high-cost curative health services, which were designed more to maximise providers' profits than to meet affiliates' basic health needs. Over-reliance on high-technology interventions and expensive imported drugs and equipment was exacerbated by the artificial over-valuation of the domestic currency between the late 1970s and early 1980s, and right through the 1990s. At the same time, there was a misguided and over-ambitious approach to service provision in the public hospitals. This devoted disproportionate levels of funding to a few state-of-the-art facilities, whilst ignoring the provision of adequate salaries, the maintenance of existing hospitals and basic primary healthcare services. The pattern of service provision in both the insurance and the public sectors was reflected in the distribution of human resources, with an extreme over-supply of doctors and shortages of qualified nursing staff. By the late 1980s there were almost five working doctors to every nurse (in developed countries the ratio is usually three nurses to every doctor). This served both to further distort service provision and to deflect funds from more cost-effective uses.

The emphasis of high cost services belied the fact that many Argentines were still without even the most primitive healthcare provision. This was reflected in the country's basic health indicators and the continued presence of many easily preventable illnesses. By the early 1990s, infant mortality rates in Argentina were higher than in Chile or Costa Rica, despite higher per capita wealth and a larger overall healthcare spend. Moreover, there was tremendous variety between rich and poor provinces, with Formosa suffering 49.1 child deaths per thousand live births in 1988, compared to only 19.9 in Buenos Aires. By the early 1990s immunisation coverage for

---

[28] Pan American Health Organisation (1995b).

conditions such as measles was well below the Latin American average, and diseases such as TB, cholera, Chagas' and even leprosy remained serious public health problems.[29] It was increasingly apparent that the existing arrangements were both highly inefficient and were failing to guarantee adequate health services for large sections of the population.

The Menem reforms

In the early 1990s the neoliberal government of Carlos Menem began to develop plans for a complete overhaul of the healthcare system. The World Bank took a large interest and, with a view to obtaining loans, was invited to provide its own studies and recommendations. From the outset, it was apparent that the reforms of health insurance and of public provision were viewed as two completely separate issues. As under previous regimes, talk of insurance reform provoked hostility from the union sector and considerable political resistance. It was seen to be strongly linked with the government's central project of promoting flexible labour markets, increasing competivity and strengthening local capital markets.[30] Conversely, public healthcare reform was not the subject of such controversy and received much less public attention, despite growing concern about those social groups who were excluded from the current economic model.

The possibility of unifying the *obra social* and public healthcare sectors was never raised either by the government, the World Bank or other international agencies. While the World Bank had examined the health sector as a whole in its 1987 study, its 1990s research gave rise to separate reports, plans and recommendations for each sector. The principal reform objectives it identified were: (i) to develop greater competition and more effective regulation of health insurance; and (ii) to improve management methods in decentralised public sector hospitals. Additional reforms for the public healthcare sector were developed with funding from the IADB. These took no account of the changes to health insurance. Indeed, the identification of respective spheres of involvement for the two development banks reflected a strong overall measure of coordination and consensus about the nature of the reform process.[31] This consensus — that health insurance and public sector reforms were essentially separate issues — also extended to key parts of the Menem government as well as the UNDP.[32]

The ultimate objective of the health insurance reforms was to merge private companies with the *obras sociales* to form a unified, competitive system. The principal reason for this was to increase 'efficiency' within the insurance sector and, it was claimed, facilitate equity through greater con-

[29] Stillwaggon (1998).

[30] Lloyd-Sherlock (1997).

[31] The 1996 World Bank report acknowledged that it was produced in close collaboration with the IADB.

[32] Although the UNDP is not providing significant funds, it is playing a strong advisory role in the reforms.

sumer choice.[33] The reforms were to be implemented in several stages. They began with measures designed to liberalise and clarify contract negotiations between union funds and private providers. Legislation enacted in 1991 and 1993 gave funds the freedom to negotiate contracts on an individual basis, rather than through collective agreements with provider associations.[34] From November 1996 a new Obligatory Medical Programme (OMP) defined a minimum set of health services (with an estimated cost of US$40 per person per month) which all the *obras sociales* were to provide. Those that were unable to meet these criteria were to be merged with others or forced to cease operations. From the start of 1997 affiliates were to be given the right to chose which *obra social* they belonged to. Finally, in January 1998 private insurance firms were to be permitted to compete for affiliates on an equal footing with the *obras sociales*, on the condition that they agreed to work within a common regulatory framework. This final phase of the reform was blocked and could not be implemented before 1999 presidential elections.

To finance the conversion of the *obras sociales* into a fully competitive system, the Health Ministry was loaned US$150 million from the World Bank and US$210 million from the treasury. To qualify to operate in the new system (and to receive part of the loan) each *obra social* had to fulfil a range of criteria. This included a requirement that the funds contain a minimum of 10,000 affiliates. Also, funds were obliged to present reports to the government containing a full financial review of the previous year's activities and a business plan. If fulfilled, this requirement would have enabled for the first time ever the compilation of a detailed database on the health insurance sector and would have greatly facilitated planning and regulation. However, by the start of 1997 only 66 of the 220 potentially eligible *obras sociales* had produced reports and only 24 of these were deemed satisfactory by the government.[35] Just four of the funds that had satisfied the reform criteria were immediately granted the loans and there appears to have been a certain degree of political discretion in the allocation of the World Bank money. Although full details about the distribution of funds have not been made available, it is apparent that most *obras* singled out for support were run by unions that supported the reforms and were closely allied to the ruling party. A typical example is the Petrol Workers' Fund (OSPE), whose union was the first to publicly support the possible re-election of Carlos Menem in 1999. As such, the process contributed to a strategy of divide and rule of the trade unions as a means of overcoming resistance to the reforms.

After apparent success in the previous stages, the Menem administration was unable to push through the final phase of the reform. There were several reasons for this failure. First, the initial reform stages were not sufficiently effective. By late 1997 it was clear that many *obras sociales* had failed to develop a

---

[33] González García and Tobar (1997).
[34] Belmartino and Bloch (1998).
[35] By mid-1998 the total number which had received funding was 29.

guaranteed basic health package for all affiliates and that even those *obras* which had benefited from substantial grants would be in no position to compete with private insurers. Indeed, it seems fair to question the wisdom of expecting the *obras* to transform themselves in the space of a single year. Also, serious defeats for the Menemist alliance in mid-term elections strengthened the position of opponents to the reform, including anti-government unions. At the same time, private insurers were already finding alternative means of entering the *obra social* sector that would leave them less subject to legal and regulatory constraints. Consequently, they no longer supported the reform proposal. The opposition of private operators to regulation was particularly significant, since the minister of health himself had a range of private interests.

Despite this setback, the central objective of the final reform stage was actually being achieved, albeit in a highly disordered and unregulated fashion. Initially in anticipation of open competition, several *obras sociales* began to foster informal ties with private insurance firms, and even when it became clear that the last phase of the reform would not be implemented, these links continued to develop. Both partners had a common interest in collaboration: to gain access to the *obras'* existing client bases and to benefit from private sector commercial expertise. As membership of an *obra social* remained obligatory, any private insurance had to be taken out in addition to *obra* cover, putting private firms at a strong competitive disadvantage. In a Trojan horse strategy known as 'triangulation', *obras sociales* began to contract out their administrative functions and increasingly served as fronts for private firms. Following the legislation for stage two of the reform, these entities were able to attract affiliates from other *obras sociales*. By December 1997 around 80 private insurers, many from the USA and Chile, had 'triangulated' with smaller *obras sociales*, which then saw a very rapid growth in membership, usually targeting high income groups.[36] This process threatened to create a new insurance hybrid which would dominate the market. The new scenario was particularly attractive to private insurers, who were able to break into the *obra social* market without being subject to any regulation.

As such, partly through legislation and partly through turning a blind eye to what were essentially illegal links between *obras* and private firms, the Menem government was able to break the deadlock of preceding decades and brought about a fundamental change in the health insurance industry. However, whether these changes would promote efficiency and equity is quite another matter. If implemented in a controlled fashion, breaking the old monopolies of the *obra sociales* and merging them with the private sector might have done much to promote efficiency. Unfortunately, this was far from the case, and control and regulation of the health insurance sector became, if anything, even worse than before the reform. Lacking transparaency and accountability, the private insurance sector was open to abuse and the system increasingly resembled the US model.

---

[36] For example, membership of the newly triangulated sea captain's *obra* grew by more than seven-fold during 1997. ('El injusto régimen de obras sociales', *La Nación* online, 30 June 1998).

There are few indications that the reform has done anything to increase equity. A small number of elite funds for groups such as senior civil servants were allowed to continue functioning much as they did before. More significantly, the new insurers developed niche strategies, attracting clients from particular employment backgrounds and with different incomes and health risks. Within this, there has been a strong bias towards providing services for richer groups. Potential profits are much higher for providing services beyond the basic OMP package to a priveleged clientele. Theoretically, a revamped redistribution fund should refund insurers if an affiliate's monthly contribution falls short of the amount required for the OMP. However, past experience shows that any redistributive mechanism is unlikely to work smoothly and this has discouraged most insurers from providing for the lower end of the market.[37] As a result, most insurers now compete for high income affiliates and, to a much more limited extent, other funds provide 'cheap and cheerful' services for the less affluent. There is little in the regulatory framework to prevent this sort of niche-seeking strategy.[38] As a result, the old system of rich and poor funds is set to continue, albeit on a rather more competitive basis. This process is already in evidence. Of the 362,332 affiliates who changed fund during 1997, the majority chose small funds that were openly specialising in services for high income clients.[39] By contrast, it recently came to light that the main *obra social* for rural workers (a clientele which are likely to appeal to private firms) had been forced to suspend most of its services because of financial problems.

However, the main failure of the reform was that no attempt was made to reduce the divide between the insurance and the public healthcare systems. It might have been hoped that greater efficiency in the new insurance system would reduce contribution levies and so facilitate access for poorer workers. This assumes that any nominal gains in efficiency would not be lost due to sales and marketing expenditure and excess profiteering. However, levies remain at exactly the same level as before the reform (three per cent for workers, five per cent for employers). The 1997 World Bank report briefly mentions logistical problems of extending insurance to the poor under the new system, observing that:

> The problems of transition to a full demand subsidy, giving the poor
> the same choice of insurer and provider as the already insured, are

---

[37] Confidence in the new redistribution fund was not helped by a decision to retain the director of its predecessor organisation, which had been widely criticised as corrupt and incompetent.

[38] In theory, insurers will not be at liberty to refuse anyone who wishes to join them, regardless of their income, age or health status and ability to make the required contributions. However, the legislation does not oblige funds to have a minimum or maximum quota of affiliates from particular groups. It is probable that a combination of targeted marketing and the erection of indirect obstacles against less attractive groups will provide the basis of an effective creamskimming strategy.

[39] *Clarín Digital* (8 Oct. 1997).

formidable. However, this could have a great potential impact on the neediest part of the population.[40]

The implication is that inclusion of the poor is a lofty ideal, out of reach for the present but which may be returned to at some unspecified future date.

As such, it is probable that a large and increasing proportion of the population would become entirely dependent on the non-insurance health sector. What reforms are being implemented here? Two initiatives have been developed with funding from the World Bank and the national government: the Nutrition Programme for Mothers and Children (PROMIN) and the Self-Managed Public Hospitals Programme (PRESSAL) Together, these programmes were allotted funding of US$475 million.[41]

The main objectives of PROMIN, which was initiated in 1992, have been to reduce levels of infant morbidity and death, strengthen primary care networks, improve pre-natal care and reduce the unnecessary use of local health centres.[42] No detailed assessments of the programme's impact are available yet, which is surprising, given its scale and the period it has been in operation. In the absence of such information, only indirect indicators can be used. Table 8.2 shows recent trends for infant mortality rates in the four provinces where this was highest at the start of the programme. This shows that significant falls were only recorded in two of these provinces. PROMIN appears to have had little impact in Formosa, whereas the dramatic improvements seen in Chaco during the 1980s were followed by a slight worsening of the situation.[43]

Table 8.2: Infant Mortality Rates per 1,000 Live Births for Selected Argentine Provinces, 1980–96

	1980	1990	1992	1996
Formosa	38.1	33.2	32.3	31.4
Chaco	54.2	35.8	33.5	34.4
Jujuy	51.4	35.8	32.5	24.4
Salta	52.1	35.8	32.8	25.5

Source: INDEC (1995), p. 165; Justo (1998), p. 76.

---

[40] World Bank (1997), p. 44.
[41] Inter-American Development Bank (IADB, 1998).
[42] *Ibid.*
[43] Infant mortality rates reflect a large number of effects and so the data in Table 8.2 should be

PRESSAL builds on a process of decentralisation begun in 1993, when a decree law offered all public hospitals the opportunity to become financially autonomous. Most of these took the opportunity, although many did not meet the quality criteria specified for inclusion. The main impact of the change was that public hospitals were able to recoup a small proportion of costs from insurance funds whose clients were using their facilities. PRESSAL itself began in 1995 and aims to give individual hospitals the right to contract personnel, administer their own budgets, recover costs from insurers and, it is claimed, introduce more cost-effective management structures. It is argued that this could benefit poorer groups through the development of effective information and financial systems in hospitals to facilitate the targeting of spending to the needy, prevent the abuse of user fees and retrieve costs for providing care to insured people.

The programme began with pilot schemes in 15 hospitals in Greater Mendoza and the Federal Capital districts. These were initiated in 1997, and, despite the fact that no systematic evaluation has yet been carried out, it is planned that they will lay the ground for a nationwide reform from 1999. The choice of the Federal Capital and Mendoza as sites for the initial PRESSAL studies is questionable. These are two of the richest parts of the country and there are strong indications that their health services are already better funded and managed than many of the poorer provinces. As such, success in these areas may not be replicable at the national level. Moreover, hospitals that have not been included in the initial pilot phase will not receive comparable levels of financial and logistical support. The process of decentralisation requires major changes in skills and managerial culture not unlike those faced by enterprises in formerly centrally planned economies. Without large-scale support, it is likely that public hospital services will face serious disruption. More importantly, there is little hard evidence that the delegation of financial control to hospitals has led to overall benefits in equity in other countries or even in Argentina.[44] Decentralisation may have sat well with the neoliberal credo of the Menem government and overseas agencies, but should not be advocated as a magic bullet for hospitals' financial problems until more is known.

A second set of public healthcare reforms valued at US$300 million was recently developed by the national government in conjunction with the IADB (which is loaning half of the projected cost). These seek to comple-

---

interpreted with extreme caution. Also, it should be remembered that data collected in poor districts of the Argentine interior are not always of the highest quality.

[44] Cassels (1995) expresses concern about the dearth of empirical studies of healthcare reform in developing countries. In one of the few detailed surveys carried out in Latin America, González-Block et al. (1989) found that decentralising healthcare administration in poor Mexican provinces often led to a reduction in equity. One of the very few public hospitals in Argentina which has a long experience of self-managament is the flagship childrens' hospital in Buenos Aires, but even here there were still problems of recouping costs from *obras sociales* and on a visit to the hospital the author found indications that patients with health insurance received preferential treatment. It is unlikely that less prestigious hospitals with fewer resources and skills would fare any better.

ment and consolidate the PRESSAL and PROMIN projects. The reforms are mainly concerned with improving the human resources of the healthcare system and directing them away from specialist curative care. This will include retraining specialists as general practitioners and the establishment of integrated health teams involving doctors, nurses and social workers. Smaller sums will be devoted to improving basic infrastructure and 'social communication' (an activity which is as much concerned with marketing policy as with educating about health). Four provinces were selected for the first phase of the reform, to take effect from the start of 1999, with a second set were to be selected for the following year.[45]

The PROMIN, PRESSAL and IADB reform measures contain some positive elements but have left many important issues unresolved. First, no direct reference is made by either the World Bank or the IADB to the widespread and often abusive practice of levying user fees and copayments within the public sector. It is not possible to obtain even rough estimates about the scale of these payments, although they are thought to be widespread.[46] Second, no concerted effort is being made to reduce the oversupply of doctors to the healthcare system. Indeed, with the proliferation of private universities offering new degrees in medicine, it is expected that there will be a sharp increase in the total number of medics. Increasing the proportion of generalists may partly mitigate this, but does not address the underlying issue: too many doctors and not enough nurses. However, the two most important shortcomings of the public healthcare reforms are that they are completely dissociated from changes in the insurance sector and that they will not entail funding increases which are anywhere near large enough to address the sector's many problems: decrepit hospitals, obsolete equipment and woefully underpaid staff. These two failings are closely linked. The deepening segmentation of the healthcare system will further drain the public sector of resources and weaken any calls to upgrade it radically. Public provision will increasingly become the refuge of poor and vulnerable groups. And, as is widely recognised by healthcare experts, ' ... a service for the poor is a poor service'.[47]

Healthcare reforms under the new administration.

In December 1999 Menem's Peronist Party lost the general election to a centrist coalition, known as the Alianza, ending more than a decade of rule. Healthcare reform had not figured prominently in the election campaign, in comparison with concerns about macroeconomic stability and corruption.[48] There was uncertainty about the future of the reform process under the Alianza, which had made no mention of an alternative project during the campaign. However, within months of taking office

---

[45] IADB (1998).
[46] Katz and Muñoz (1988).
[47] Abel-Smith (1994).
[48] Tedesco (2000).

the new administration had been able to succeed where Menem had failed: pushing through by decree the final phase of the health insurance reform, which allows private funds to compete freely with the *obras sociales*. In return, private funds are to be subject to state regulation and are to be obliged to provide the full Obligatory Medical Package without discrimination on the basis of age, income or pre-existing conditions. The new arrangement will take effect from January 2001.

The completion of the Menemist health insurance project was expected to generate widespread popular support from key Alianza constituencies. By the late 1990s, private health insurance had extended its reach to a significant number of middle class Argentines.[49] Most of these were also obliged to pay *obra social* contributions, and so the new system should reduce their overall monthly payments. The Alianza's strategy may have also reflected the recognition that competition between private and *obra social* funds was already occurring on an informal basis, and that it would be difficult to end. Moreover, the new administration was in a better position to push through the reform than the Peronists had been in the run-up to the election. The Alianza had a strong popular mandate and had fewer historical ties with trades unions.

The completion of the Menemist project might be interpreted as a missed opportunity to reconsider the general direction that healthcare reform was taking in Argentina. Nevertheless, a half-complete reform would have represented an even worse option, giving private firms free rein to operate in a chaotic, unregulated marketplace. The key to the reform's success will be the capacity of state agencies to carry out their regulatory functions. The Alianza has placed great emphasis on improving governance: effective supervision of the new healthcare system will be a stiff test of its mettle.

Conclusions

It is impossible to understand the current structure and reforms of Argentina's healthcare system without reference to its development over the past hundred years or so. The historical review sketched out in the first part of the chapter shows that there was a striking degree of continuity of institutional arrangements, particularly in the health insurance sector. Throughout the period studied, health insurance remained separate from the provision and financing of public healthcare services. Insurance funds covered a large section of the formal workforce, they were usually structured along occupational lines, mainly administered by unions and extremely heterogeneous. Likewise, the public health system remained a 'poor relation' throughout the century, usually suffering from chronic under-funding and from political wrangling between different tiers of government. If past regimes had been singularly unsuc-

---

[49] Data for private health insurance membership do not exist.

cessful in altering the basic structure of the healthcare system, it is fair to question what real impact the current health reforms may have.

The reforms of the Menem and Alianza administrations have broken with the past trends by ending the old monopolies of the *obras sociales*. This has been a major achievement and it could have laid the basis for a fundamental restructuring of the healthcare system. It was made possible by a range of factors, including the intervention of the World Bank, which provided essential financing and the means to coopt key trade unions. The unions themselves had become weaker political actors over time, due to deindustrialisation and changes to labour legislation. The insurance reform was also facilitated by the broader neoliberal changes that had been occurring in Argentina since 1989 and laid the foundations for a scaled-down, but aggressive, private insurance sector which was keen to compete with the *obras sociales*. As a result, for the first time Argentines are now able to select which insurance fund they participate in. This will inevitably lead to the disappearance of the smaller and less efficient *obras sociales*. However, it is likely that the quality of care offered by funds will remain variable, due to niche marketing and cream skimming. There are no clear signs that any of the other health insurance reform measures, particularly those involving regulation, have been effectively implemented. Many *obras sociales* still fail to offer the basic medical package or to supply the official monitor with up-to-date information. With the encroachment of private insurers, the industry has become increasingly unregulated and unaccountable.

Many of the reforms proposed for the public health sector look promising on paper, but there has been little assessment of those already initiated and there are many potential barriers to effective implementation. Also, existing proposals leave a number of key issues unaddressed. As a result, it is likely that a bias towards high-cost interventions instead of ensuring basic services for all will largely survive. Consequently, the reforms will not lead to major changes in the historical pattern of under-funded, overly curative public healthcare.

Taken as a whole, the current reforms' greatest shortcoming is their failure to develop a global healthcare system meeting the needs of the entire population. Around 35 per cent or more of Argentines will remain outside the health insurance system and will continue to rely on a public sector strapped for funds and in which little significant change is likely to occur. Given long-term labour market trends of greater informalisation and unemployment, it is likely that this excluded group will increase in size. As such, the reforms of recent years can be characterised as a missed opportunity to develop a truly efficient, equitable and universal healthcare system.

CHAPTER 9

Health Reform and Equity in Colombia

Francisco Yepes

Introduction

This chapter presents the equity conditions of the Colombian health system before and after the last wave of reforms. After a brief discussion of the general background, the previous system is described, as well as the decentralisation (1990) and the social security (1993) reforms. Health system equity in terms of outcomes, allocation of resources, insurance coverage before the reforms and insurance coverage after the 1993 reform are presented.

Although Colombia, a constitutional multi-party democracy, has had a relatively 'stable' political system with uninterrupted elected governments for most of this century, it has been in a state of internal war for more than 50 years. This aggravates problems of governability and affects the government's ability to introduce reform. The civil population is caught in the crossfire of the main war actors: guerrillas, paramilitary groups, peasant self-defence forces and government armed forces. More than 1,300,000 war refugees are living in very inadequate conditions. For the last decade, the total number of homicides has been over 25,000 per year and 25 per cent of the total burden of disease is attributable to homicides, a far greater proportion than for the world (one per cent) or Latin America as a whole (three per cent).[1]

Colombia is a lower middle income country, with 36.8 million inhabitants, 73 per cent urban, 91 per cent literate. It has a GDP of US$1910 (at 1995 exchange rate), life expectancy of 70 years, infant mortality of 26 per 1,000, maternal mortality of 107 per 100,000 and total fertility rate of 2.8. Among the countries of Latin America it ranks third in population, fifth in geographical size and ninth in per capita GNP (see Table 9.1). Its epidemiological profile presents a coexistence of communicable and chronic diseases with trauma from motor vehicle accidents and violence. In 1994 Colombia lost 5,512,686 Disability-Adjusted Life Years (DALYs),[2] 57 per cent of them corresponding to premature mortality and 43 per cent due to disability from different causes. Thirty-nine per cent of DALYs were due to trauma from violence and motor vehicle accidents, 39 per cent attributable to non-communicable diseases and 22 per cent to communicable diseases.[3]

---

[1] Ministerio de Salud (1994).
[2] DALY is a measure that combines years of life lost due to premature death and reduction in quality of life due to disability.
[3] Ministerio de Salud (1994).

Table 9.1: Colombia's Standing among other Latin-American Countries

Country	Population (1)	Population in poverty (2)	Urban Population (3)	Infant Mortality (4)	Maternal Mortality (5)	Life expectancy (6)
Brazil	161.7	50	78	57	140	66.3
Argentina	34.5	25	88	26	52	72.1
Mexico	91.1	40	75	30	45	71.5
Colombia	**35.1**	**37**	**73**	**32**	**140**	**69.3**
Peru	23.7	52	72	59	261	66.0
Cuba	11.0	—	76	10	32	75.3
Costa Rica	3.4	24	50	12	40	76.3

Source: Pan American Health Organisation, Basic Health Indicators (1995)
(1) In thousands, 1995
(2) Per cent, between 1990 and 1994
(3) Per cent, 1995
(4) Per 1,000 live births, 1994
(5) Per 100,000 live births, 1987 and 1993
(6) At birth, 1990–95

Colombia's health system has its roots in pre-Columbian times as well as in its Spanish inheritance, enriched through time with influences from Bismarck's Germany, the French and United States' medical schools and the PAHO/CENDES planning model, [4] among others. Although, from colonial times there have been government agencies responsible for the different health activities, the country had to wait until 1946 to have the first free-standing Ministry of Hygiene, later called the Ministry of Public Health and more recently the Ministry of Health. That same year the Social Security Institute (Instituto de Seguros Sociales) which offered a Bismarckian social security insurance scheme to private sector workers, and an equivalent for public workers at national level (Caja Nacional de Previsión) were also instituted. [5] Over the years the social security subsector evolved to include more than 100 different social security institutions covering public workers at departmental and municipal levels. Together, they covered 23.8 per cent of the population, with the Institute of Social Security covering 11.3 per cent and the others accounting for the remaining 12.5 per cent. [6] The latter were social security institutions for public workers at the departmental and municipal levels, for Congress, for the Ministry of Communications and

---

[4] The PAHO/CENDES model was a health planning model developed in the 1960s and it was very much in use in the health sector at that time. It based the definition of priorities on a mathematical formula based on criteria of mortality, morbidity, vulnerability and social values.
[5] Avila (1988).
[6] Ruiz and Torres (1990).

even for local hospitals. Most of these were small and quite inefficient institutions, providing both retirement and health benefits.

The Colombian health system has been reformed several times in the course of this century, following the prevailing conceptions of the state and the influence of international organisations.[7] In the latter half of the 1970s, a National Health System was created, with a highly centralised structure and a powerful Ministry of Health at its apex.

The system, which existed before the last round of reforms, consisted of three tiers. A *private subsector* served mainly, but not exclusively, the affluent classes, who either had private insurance schemes or paid on a fee-for-service basis. There was a *social security* scheme, which never achieved more than 25 per cent coverage and was mainly concentrated in the largest urban areas. Affiliates included workers of the formal sector and national, departmental and municipal public employees who contributed eight per cent of their salary (one third from the worker and two thirds from the employer). Lastly, a *public sector* with hospitals, health centres and health posts served the poor and uninsured. The government admitted that 20 per cent of the population was not reached by any subsector.

The social security health services served only the insured, but the insured population did not necessarily limit their use of health services to the social security institutions. The insured population in the upper income groups would never use the social security health services or would use them only in case of expensive treatments. Multiple coverage with compulsory social insurance plus private insurance or employer provided services was not an uncommon practice.

The public sector owned 63.5 per cent of the hospitals, plus approximately 3,000 health centres and posts. The social security sector owned 4.9 per cent of hospitals, most of them through the Social Security Institute, and the private sector 31.7 per cent of hospitals. Health professionals could work in either subsector or in several of them.

Within the public sector, there were three administrative levels: the Ministry of Health at the National level; the Department of Health services at the department level and the local health services at the municipal level. The Ministry of Health set the policies, defined the programmes, established the financing, actually carried out several services, nominated the Department of Health secretaries and supervised. The Department of Health Secretariats were mainly intermediary coordinating agencies and the local (municipal) services were in charge of the actual provision of services, through community hospitals, health centres and posts. The latter were wholly run from the department level with no participation of the municipal administration whatsoever, except in some large cities (see Figure 9.1 for a scheme of the system).

---

[7] Quevedo (1990).

Figure 9.1: The Colombian Health System before the 1990/1993 Reforms

Ministry of Health (Set policies, norms and regulations; supervise, provide services)		
33 Department health services (supervise, coordinate and provide services)	**Institute of Social Security and more than 100 social security institutions** (insure and provide services)	**Private hospitals, laboratories, physicians** (sell services)
Municipal hospitals, centres and posts (wholly run by the department, provide services)		
Official subsector (public)	**Social security (public)**	**Private subsector**

The pre-reform healthcare system suffered from a number of serious prob-lems. First, there were important inefficiencies.[8] By the early 1990s Colombia was already spending over seven per cent of its GNP on health, but the results were poor compared to other Latin American countries with similar spending levels. This was partly because the system was extremely centralised, with many operational decisions made at Ministry of Health level (for example, hospital budgets, hospital payrolls). Concentration on operational problems distracted the ministry from policy formulation and monitoring, and high centralisation detached local communities from their health services. Priorities allocated at the national level did not necessarily reflect local needs.

There were also problems of equity. Health insurance levels never reached beyond 24 per cent, with insurance schemes limited to the workers, with no coverage for their families except pregnant wives and children un-der one year of age. The rest of the population either paid for private health services or utilised public ones. In 1988 it was estimated that per capita health expenditures for the workers affiliated to the Social Security Institute were seven times those of the poor, taken care of by the Ministry of Health. Access to health services favoured the rich and the social security affiliates. Hospitalisation rates for higher income groups were almost double those of the lower income ones and those of the social security affiliates were more than double those of the non-affiliated.[9]

There were clear differences between geographical regions in terms of levels of insurance coverage. Table 9.2 shows how Bogotá had more than double the coverage of any other region and triple that of the Atlantic region. Intra-regional differences were also important, to the point of there being a

---

[8] Yepes (1990a).
[9] Yepes (1990b).

five-fold difference in government per capita health expenditures between the department getting the least funds and the one getting the most.

Table 9.2: Insurance Coverage by Region. Colombia 1986–89

Region	Per cent insurance coverage
Atlantic	16.5
Eastern	18.9
Central	20.0
Pacific	23.4
Bogotá	49.4

Source: Escuesta Nacional sobre CAP's en salud (1986–89). *Seguridad Social*, vol 1. *Características de la población* (Ministerio de Salud, Instituto Nacional de Salud, Instituto de Seguros Sociales).

Inequities in service provision partly explain the high degree of geographical variation observed for various key indicators of health status. There are important regional and urban/rural differentials in infant mortality, with the highest mortality figures in the least developed parts of the country — the Pacific littoral and the south-east.[10] Moreover, studies have found that malnutrition is significantly higher among the less educated and the less affluent.[11]

The reforms

Starting in the late 1980s, there have been two main sets of reforms in the health system. The first set centred on the **decentralisation** of health services to the municipal levels, as part of a general decentralisation of the state. This strategy has been immersed in an effort to modernise the state administration, making it more efficient and strengthening democracy through widened citizens' participation in the planning, management and control of municipal life.[12]

After several unsuccessful decentralising efforts which date from 1945, a series of acts started a profound decentralisation effort throughout the whole administration: Acts 14 of 1983, 11 and 12 of 1986 and a series of decrees, 77,

---

[10] Yepes (1990a).
[11] Mora (1982).
[12] Manrique and Marín (1987).

78, 79, 80 and 91 of 1987,[13] which paved the way for a comprehensive decentralisation process with political, administrative and fiscal components, incorporated as a constitutional mandate in the new Constitution of 1991.

Figure 9.2: The Colombian Health System after the 1990/1993 Reforms

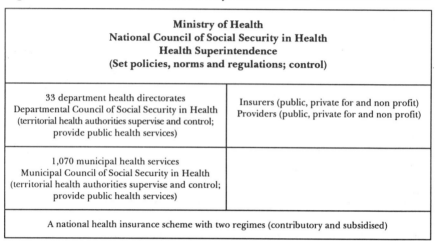

Ministry of Health National Council of Social Security in Health Health Superintendence (Set policies, norms and regulations; control)	
33 department health directorates Departmental Council of Social Security in Health (territorial health authorities supervise and control; provide public health services)	Insurers (public, private for and non profit) Providers (public, private for and non profit)
1,070 municipal health services Municipal Council of Social Security in Health (territorial health authorities supervise and control; provide public health services)	
A national health insurance scheme with two regimes (contributory and subsidised)	

Political decentralisation involved the actual transfer of power to the departmental and municipal territories through the popular election of department governors and municipal mayors. *Administrative* decentralisation occurred through the redefinition of roles and responsibilities of the federal government, departments and municipalities with the latter assuming many responsibilities that were before in the hands of the federal government or the department. The construction of rural roads, schools, hospitals, health centres and posts, water supply and sewage systems — which were previously managed directly by several national institutes — was transferred to the municipalities and the institutes were closed. Finally, *fiscal* decentralisation saw the actual transfer of economic resources to carry out the new responsibilities. Transfers to the municipalities rose from 4.3 per cent of the GNP in 1990 to 7.7 per cent in 1997.

Health decentralisation was mainly set by Act 10 of 1990 and was complemented by Act 60 of 1993. Municipalities, which before decentralisation did not have any responsibility in the health system, now became major actors. The municipal mayors are now the heads of the municipal health system. They are obliged to develop a local health plan, which would be integrated into the general municipal one, and they are responsible for the health of their communities either through the direct provision of health services, or contracting with public or private providers and developing public health activities. This policy intended to make the local health services sensitive to local health needs, by developing health plans,

---

[13] *Ibid.*

setting local health priorities, performing local health programming and encouraging the community to participate in all phases. This has been achieved to varying degrees across the country.[14]

The second set of reforms was that of the **social security system**, which reflected changes in the role of the state in the face of economic opportunities and globalisation trends. Act 100 of 1993, as a development of the new 1991 Constitution, established a National Health Insurance scheme with the goal of attaining universal coverage by the year 2001. This Act significantly transformed the health sector and introduced new actors and practices into the system (see Figure 9.3). It established the basis of the reform, setting five guiding principles: efficiency, universality, solidarity, comprehensiveness and social participation.

Figure 9.3: The Colombian Health System

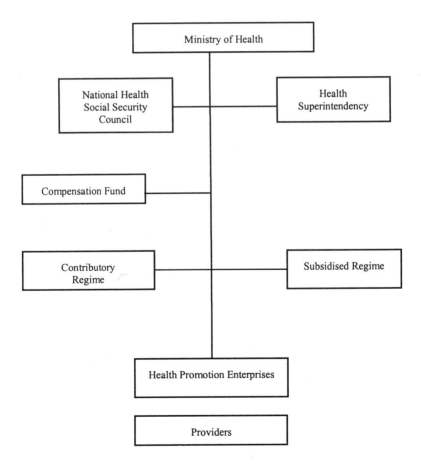

---

[14] Yepes, Sánchez and Castor (1999).

Efficiency

The reform seeks to promote efficiency by managed competition and free choice of insurer. A two-tiered system of managed competition has been created in which private and public, for profit and not-for-profit insurers compete in the market to offer a government-set standard health benefit package, and on the other hand, providers compete to sell their services to insurers. For their part, consumers are free to select an insurer and to select providers of services from those with a contract with their insurer. They have the right to change insurer once a year.

Universality

Universality is sought through compulsory social insurance with family coverage, funded by employer/employee contributions and by government subsidies. There are two ways of accessing the social insurance system. The contributory regime is for those with a formal labour contract irrespective of their income level and for self-employed workers earning more than two minimum wages. They contribute 12 per cent of their income (eight per cent from the employer and four per cent from the employee; the self-employed are responsible for the full amount). It is estimated that 70 per cent of the population will fall into this regime. Contributions are collected by the insurers (called Empresas Promotoras de Salud — EPSs) who get paid by a risk adjusted premium (capitation) in such a way that a particular insurer, depending on the income/risk mix of affiliates, may generate a surplus or deficit in its actual premium collection. The law has established a compensation fund where the insurers (EPSs) either deposit their excess collections or are reimbursed for their deficits.

The subsidised regime is for the poor. It is estimated that 30 per cent of the population will be covered by this regime. Municipal mayors are responsible for identifying the poor through the application of a targeting instrument (means test) which classifies the poor into three levels of poverty. Level 1, the poorest of the poor, will get a 95 per cent subsidy, level 2 a 90 per cent subsidy and level 3 a 70 per cent subsidy.

All persons, in either regime, will select an EPS that will be responsible for the provision of a standard health benefit package. EPSs may provide the required services through their own (but administratively distinct) network of providers or through contracted ones. Besides the EPSs, and exclusively for the subsidised regime, the law allows the presence of other insurers which do not have such stringent requirements as the EPSs, are not-for-profit and in many instances are of community origin. These are called Subsidised Regime Administrators.

The law allows the development of complementary health packages, which can be purchased by anybody, willing and able to pay extra for additional coverage or better amenities.

Solidarity

There are at least three solidarity mechanisms in the system. First, the contributory system has its own internal solidarity, since those earning more subsidise those earning less.[15] Second, one per cent of the contributory regime payments is assigned by law to cross-subsidise the poor of the subsidised regime. Third, the subsidised regime is financed from general taxation.

Comprehensiveness

By setting a standard health benefits package, the government establishes comprehensive coverage of preventive and curative services, which all insurers must offer. Subsidised membership provides a less comprehensive benefits package. Starting at 50 per cent coverage of the contributory benefit package, it should increase through time as resources permit. In fact it is now around 60 per cent. Both packages (subsidised and contributory) should include health promotion and preventive care. Furthermore, insurers are not allowed to deny cover to anyone applying for insurance and exclusion of pre-existing conditions is prohibited so as to avoid adverse selection practices.

Social participation

Acts 10 of 1990, 100 of 1993 and the 1991 Constitution explicitly laid down mechanisms and means for social participation and social control. Consumers may, at will, become constituted in consumer alliances at the level of insurers or providers and citizen surveillance bodies must be created to control public investment. The law established a National Health Social Security Council as a central coordinating body for the system, with representation from the government, insurers, providers, professionals and community. This council sets the content of the standard benefit packages and the level of the capitation provided to insurers. It also established a compensation fund that manages all the resources of the contributory regime. A consortium of accounting firms administers this fund. They act as fiduciary agent with four internal sub accounts: one to collect the surpluses from the EPSs and to redistribute to those with deficits; a second corresponding to the one per cent cross subsidy for the poor; a third for the promotion and prevention programmes of EPSs; and the fourth for catastrophic events and traffic accidents.

The law also reformed the National Health Superintendency, enabling it to monitor the system and in particular its financial and quality aspects. Furthermore, it set the framework for the transition from supply financing to demand financing for public hospitals. In order to prepare for competition with the private sector, they are to be transformed into State Social Enterprises with legal, administrative and financial autonomy and modernised management.

---

[15] The contribution of an individual to the contributory regime, and his family capitation which is paid to the insurer, would be equal to around 2.25 times the minimum wage for an estimated average family size of 3.64.

Under the decentralisation process, municipalities have major responsibilities for the local operation of health insurance, particularly for ensuring that the poor receive a means test and are insured. They are responsible for convening the Subsidised Regime Administrators interested in servicing the locality, paying them the corresponding capitation in accordance with the number of subsidised affiliates they insure and supervising their operations.

Implementation of the reforms

Both reforms have been difficult to implement and both are still in progress. Both have changed and will continue to change the relationships between the state, the population and the providers. Decentralisation has meant important power shifts among the territorial governments involved (nation, departments and municipalities). The national level has been freed of responsibility for the actual provision of services, allowing it to develop its role in policy formulation and technical assistance. The municipalities have assumed control over local health decisions and the departments have had their control reduced over municipal decisions. There has been both resistance and opposition from different actors, whose interests have been affected. Resistance at state level has not been uncommon and there is a lack of adequate incentives for the departments and municipalities to decentralise.[16] The institutional capacity at municipal level is still lacking, due to the complexity of the new responsibilities assumed and the lack of expertise and experience at municipal level, particularly in the small localities.

As to the social security reform, the major limitation has been the lack of experience and of adequate information. It has been a process of learning on the job in a country which had no experience with capitation payments or standard health benefit packages, and where cost information on health services was non-existent. The social security reform introduced new actors into the system, who, in many instances, had to start from scratch. The health insurers (EPSs) were totally new to the system, as were the Compensation Fund and the National Health Social Security Council. New and unfamiliar concepts were introduced. Capitation payment had not existed previously, since salary and fee-for-service had been the prevailing forms of payment. Also new were the standard health benefit packages and the change from supply to demand subsidies. Appropriate software did not exist for the needs of the new institutions, which led to buying expensive solutions in Chile and Brazil. These have proved inadequate for Colombian requirements and they have been replaced with tailor-made packages.

Most of the above problems are considered to be soluble through regulations without changing the law. There seems to be agreement on

---

[16] Vargas and Sarmiento (1997). The departments are afraid of losing power to the municipalities and resist transferring control of the hospitals to them. Since the departments get the fiscal transfers automatically, there is no way of penalising them. The municipalities also get the transfers automatically and do not have incentives to modernise their administration.

the adequacy of the macro design of the reforms[17] and on the macroeconomic viability of the system. However, several observers have pointed to problem areas that need to be addressed to avoid future complications. Some of these are developmental. New institutions were created and new concepts and processes adopted. Where there was no culture of national health insurance, there was a need to learn about the importance and the need to get insured. Where there was no tradition of capitation payment, it was necessary to learn how to contract based on capitation. The poor needed to learn the advantages of being insured and the rights derived from it, and although they did not initially utilise the services, they have learned by now. Public hospitals had to learn how to bill for their services and they are only starting to realise that the new system requires them to market their services. Development of adequate information systems has become a must.

Some problems may be less easy to solve. There is an excess of norms and regulations,[18] which diminishes the transparency of the processes and increases the difficulty of citizen control. The financing mechanisms of the subsidised regime are excessively complex and cumbersome.[19] The way that part of the government funds are allocated geographically has been identified as highly inequitable; as a result, this is not encouraging a reduction in regional differences.[20]

The process of transformation from supply to demand subsidies, which goes parallel with the transformation of public hospitals into State Social Enterprises, is moving slowly.[21] In 1996, 87 per cent of the public health resources were still assigned in the traditional way.[22] This adds difficulty to the growth of subsidised coverage, which depends in good part on this transformation. On the other hand, those public hospitals that for many years have been under the protection of the state and whose management has been below standard are in urgent need of developing modern management structures, a process that requires time.

Evasion, by non-affiliation of people who should be in the contributory regime or by under-declaration of income, has been repeatedly identified[23] and might affect the economic viability of the reform model.[24] Estimates are that 35 per cent or more of the population who should be in the contributory regime are still not affiliated, and that there is at least a 30 per cent under-declaration of income.

Public health programmes, one of the few strengths of the previous system, have been affected first by decentralisation and then by the so-

---

[17] Jaramillo et al. (1998).
[18] Vargas and Sarmiento (1997).
[19] Jaramillo et al. (1998).
[20] Vargas and Sarmiento (1997).
[21] Medina (1997).
[22] Vargas and Sarmiento (1997).
[23] Sánchez and Yepes (1997); Jaramillo et al. (1998).
[24] Giedion and Wollner (1996).

cial security reform. Municipalities have not completed the process of taking over their new responsibilities, and their information systems and epidemiological surveillance have been seriously affected.[25] An outbreak of equine meningitis in the northern part of the country went undetected until it was too late, and this has happened also with dengue fever outbreaks in the south-west.

Professional dissatisfaction is a general concern arising from several factors. There has been no strategy to prepare the professionals for the reform; financial negotiations with the insurers have not always been satisfactory; and professional autonomy has been affected by the relationship with the insurers.[26] Health professionals in general, but physicians in particular, were unprepared for a reform which drastically changed their practices: as insurance coverage increases, fewer patients come individually on a fee-for-service basis and more through the insurers on a prepaid basis. Middle-aged physicians with established practices have probably been more affected, while recent graduates now find it easier to start a professional practice.

Public information and education have been grossly insufficient and have affected people's ability to exercise their rights. During 1997 the Subsidised Regime Administrators experienced a lower than expected demand for services by their affiliates, reportedly because the insured lacked information about their rights. Since they are paid on a capitation basis and their profit margins were getting too high, they were required to use the 'excess profits' to create reserves.

Quality assurance is almost non-existent and there is no information about what might be happening with quality of care in a system under significant pressure to control costs. There are also doubts about the macro-economic efficiency of the system. The reform brought new resources to the health sector. It is estimated that by 1996, total health expenditures were at 10.1 per cent of GDP (4.2 per cent private/5.9 per cent public),[27] up from 7.0 per cent (3.9 per cent private/3.1 per cent public) before the reform.[28] Yet 50 per cent of the population remains uninsured, although half of these are still covered by the public system under the transitional arrangements.

There are population groups excluded from the system because the law has allowed special arrangements for them: the armed forces, schoolteachers and oil workers. On solidarity grounds it is considered that these exclusions should be eliminated.[29] Congressmen, who until very recently also had special status, have had this status outlawed by a provision of the State Council.

The Social Security Institute, which existed before the reform as the largest public health insurer, was allowed to remain and to become an EPS. Al-

---

[25] Jaramillo (1997).

[26] Jaramillo et al. (1998). In order to control costs, the insurers submit certain diagnostic and therapeutic procedures to prior approval and the prescription of drugs under compulsory insurance is limited to the official essential drug list.

[27] Vargas and Sarmiento (1997).

[28] Velandia et al. (1990); Harvard University School of Public Health (1996).

[29] This applies in particular to the oil workers, who are among the best paid in the country.

though it is still the largest EPS, it has been losing afiliates, decreasing its share of the market from almost 75 per cent to about 50 per cent and is in serious financial crisis because of an inherited structure of very high fixed costs.

Impact of the reforms

There have been a number of key achievements. A first major achievement has been the construction of a consensus around the social security reform. In spite of all the difficulties, all major actors agree on the need for the reform for the country and consider it a major social attainment, although many may have criticisms of specific aspects.[30]

By the end of 1997, insurance coverage was at 46.6 per cent for both regimes,[31] a figure that more than doubled what the country had been able to achieve during almost 50 years of the previous system. The subsidised regime already covered 13 per cent of the population (5,130,000), that is 43 per cent of the estimated target (30 per cent), while the contributory regime covered approximately 33 per cent of the population, up from 20 per cent before the reform. The contributory coverage increase can be explained by the introduction of family coverage, which is now compulsory. This implies that, except for the effect of the inclusion of family members, there are not many new insured under this regime. The subsidised coverage is particularly significant since it is reaching the poorer section of the population, including 65 per cent of the population with unsatisfied basic needs, and is a reflection of the priority to equity given by the government. However, regional differences persist and very large differences in insurance coverage still occur across socioeconomic groups (see Tables 9.3 and 9.4).

Table 9.3: Health Insurance Coverage by Region, Colombia, 1997

Region	Coverage %
Atlantic	43.19
Central	51.85
Pacific	56.37
Eastern	65.25
Bogotá	65.41
Antioquia	64.88
Orinoquia	69.79

Data Source: *Quality of Life Survey* (Departamento Administrativo Nacional de Estadística, 1997).

[30] Jaramillo et al. (1998).
[31] Coverage figures are estimates from different sources and not completely reliable.

Table 9.4: Insurance Coverage by Socioeconomic Stratum, Colombia, 1997

Stratum	Coverage %
Unclassified*	43.97
1	53.96
2	58.68
3	70.39
4	80.65
5	89.94
6	87.89
9**	64.53

Data Source: *Quality of Life Survey* (Departamento Administrativo Nacional de Estadística, 1997).

* Population living in municipalities with no state registration for public services or with illegal connections. It is reasonable to assume that this represents poor sectors of the population.
** Population which at the time of the survey could not document the stratum.

There are 30 EPSs[32] offering contributory insurance and approximately 231 Subsidised Regime Administrators. All municipalities in the country have at least one insurer present, 70 per cent at least two and all state capitals at least five. The Ministry of Health and the departmental health secretaries have been relieved of the responsibility for the direct provision of services, moving into activities connected with the management of the system and strengthening their policy formulation/monitoring capabilities. During 1996, the private EPSs, which contribute to the Compensation and Solidarity Fund, produced surpluses of US$88 million,[33] more than enough to compensate the two EPSs in deficit and leave reserves for future needs.

Under the old system there were captive clienteles for the Social Security Institute and the other social security institutions, where employees did not have the choice to select an insurer unless they opted to pay twice. People are now free to select their insurer and once a year they can exercise the right to move to a different one. However, the double contribution has not been eliminated, particularly for the higher socioeconomic groups who are not satisfied with the choice of provider offered by compulsory insurance and choose to buy additional packages of prepaid medicine which may in part duplicate the basic insurance cover.

---

[32] Since the beginning of the reform, two EPSs have gone out of business.
[33] The difference between the contributions of the insured and the capitation rate.

This is a problem that could be solved by government regulations setting caps on the amount the insurers can charge for complementary services.

The country still has a lot to learn in order to succeed with the new system. It is necessary to streamline norms and strengthen government institutions with improved information systems, to enforce and monitor compliance. Likewise, a very significant effort is required for a massive re-education of the human resources of the health system and extended information and education of the public on the new system.

There are various questions and concerns that are still unanswered.

- What should be the future of the public network be? Public hospitals are going through a profound change to adapt to the new system. As ordered by Act 100, they have been changing their legal status, becoming State Social Enterprises. In this way, they obtain administrative and financial autonomy, which they did not have before. At the same time, the financing they used to get from government subsidies (supply financing) is progressively drying up, to be replaced by the income they are able to get by selling their services in the market. Undoubtedly, there are incentives in place for hospitals to modernise their administration and become efficient institutions, and they are moving in this direction. However, since the law allows the insurers to own their own network of provider institutions, the question remains whether they will not move into developing these networks, particularly in the more profitable services, eventually forcing the public network out of business or buying it out.

- Will the government be able (willing) to enforce compliance with insurance, particularly for the high-income population, and control evasion? If not, the solidarity of the system and its economic viability will be seriously questioned.

- Will there be the necessary political will to correct the inequity in the distribution of government resources to regions? Poorer regions do have a larger proportion of the poor among their population and if they do not get a larger share of the transfers, they will not be able to provide subsidised insurance.

- There are questions about the role of the Social Security Institute, by far the largest EPS, which controls 50 per cent of the contributive market. The Institute does not yet know the exact number of its affiliates and there are many questions as to its financial viability in the medium term.

It is still too early in the process to answer these questions, and we will have to wait some time for answers, but it is clear that we will have to improve our ability to follow up the reform in such a way that we can provide appropriate and timely feedback to decision-makers.

Bibliography

Abel, C. and Lewis, C (eds.) (1993) *Welfare, Poverty and Development in Latin America* (London: Macmillan).

Abel-Smith, B. (1994) *An Introduction to Health. Policy, Planning and Financing* (London: Longman).

Acosta Córdova, C. and Correa, G. (1998) 'Negocia el gobierno, a espaldas del Congreso, un crédito por 700 millones de dólares para financiar la "reforma" de la seguridad social', *Proceso* no. 1117 (Mexico), March 29.

Ahumada, J. (1965) *Health Planning: Problems of Concept and Method*, PAHO Scientific Publication No. 111 (Washington, DC).

Ai Camp, R. (ed.) (1995) *Democracy in Latin America: Patterns and Cycles* (Wilmington: Scholarly Resources).

Altimir, O. (1996) *Economic Development and Social Equity: A Latin American Perspective* (Santiago de Chile: Economic Commission for Latin America and the Caribbean).

ANSAL (1994) *Health Sector Assessment Project of El Salvador. Health Sector Reform in El Salvador: Towards Equity and Efficiency. Final Report* (San Salvador: USAID).

Araujo Jr., J. (1997) 'Attempts to Decentralize in Recent Brazilian Health Policy: Issues and Problems, 1988–94', *International Journal of Health Services*, vol. 27, no. 1.

Ashton, J. and Seymour, H. (1988) *The New Public Health: The Liverpool Experience*, (Buckingham: Open University Press).

Atkinson, S. (1995) 'Restructuring Health Care: Tracking the Decentralization Debate', *Progress in Human Geography,* vol. 19, no. 4, pp. 486–503.

Atkinson, S. (1997) 'From Vision to Reality: Implementing Health Reforms in Lusaka, Zambia', *Journal of International Development*, vol. 9, no. 4, pp. 631–39

Avila, Néstor (1988) 'Historia de las instituciones de salud en Colombia', Master's thesis. Health Administration Postgraduate Programme, Javeriana University, Bogotá.

Banco Interamericano de Desarrollo (1997) *América Latina tras una década de reformas* (Washington, DC: BID).

Banerji D. (1984) 'Primary Health Care: Selective or Comprehensive', *World Forum*, no. 5:

Banta, H. (1988) 'The Transfer of Medical Technologies in Developing Countries', in F. Rutten and S. Reiser (eds.), *The Economics of Medical Technologies* (Berlin: Springer Verlag).

Barbosa, L.N. de H. (1995) 'The Brazilian *jeitinho*: An Exercise in National Identity', in D.J. Hess and R.A. Da Matta (eds.), *The Brazilian Puzzle: Culture on the Borderlands of the Western World* (New York: Columbia University Press), chapter 1, pp. 35–48.

Barrientos, A. (1998) *Pension Reform in Latin America* (Aldershot: Ashgate).

Barrientos, A. and Lloyd-Sherlock, P. (2000) 'Reforming Health Insurance in Argentina and Chile', *Health Policy and Planning*, vol. 15, no. 4, pp. 417–23.

Belmartino, S. and Bloch, C. (1982) 'Políticas sociales y seguridad social en Argentina', *Cuadernos Médico Sociales*, no. 14.

Belmartino, S. and Bloch, C. (1994) *El sector salud en Argentina. Actores, conflictos de intereses y modelos organizativos, 1960–1985* (Washington, DC: Pan American Health Organisation).

Belmartino, S. and Bloch, C. (1998) 'Desregulación/privatización: la relación entre financiación y provisión de servicios en la reforma de la seguridad social médica en Argentina', *Cuadernos Médico Sociales*, vol. 73.

Belmartino, S. et al. (1991) *Fundamentos históricos de la construcción de relaciones de poder en el sector salud. Argentina 1940–1960* (Washington, DC: Pan American Health Organisation).

Berlin, I. (1992) 'The Pursuit of the Ideal', in I. Berlin, *The Crooked Timber of Humanity.* (New York: Vintage Books), pp. 1–19.

Berry, R. (ed.) (1998) *Poverty, Economic Reform and Income Distribution in Latin America* (Boulder, London: Lynne Rienner).

BID, BIRF, CEPAL, OEA, OPS/OMS, FNUAP, UNICEF, USAID (1996) *Reunión Especial sobre Reforma del Sector Salud (29–30 de septiembre de 1995)* (Washington, DC: Pan American Health Organisation).

Blum, W. (1986) *The CIA, a Forgotten History* (London: Zed Books).

Bobadilla, J.L. (1988) *Quality of Perinatal Medical Care in Mexico City* (Mexico City: National Institute of Public Health).

Bobadilla, J.L., Frenk, J., Lozano, R., Frejka, T. and Stern, C. (1993) 'The Epidemiologic Transition and Health Priorities', in D.T. Jamison, W.H. Mosley, A.R. Measham and J.L. Bobadilla (eds.), *Disease Control Priorities in Developing Countries* (New York: Oxford University Press for the World Bank), pp. 51–63.

Bossert, T. (1995) 'Decentralization', in K. Janovsky (ed.), *Health Policy and Systems Development* (Geneva: WHO), chapter 9, pp. 147–60.

Bossert T., Hsiao, W., Barrera, M., Alarcon, L., Leo, M. and Casares, C. (1998) 'Transformation of Ministries of Health in the Era of Health Reform: The Case of Colombia', *Health Policy and Planning*, vol. 13, pp. 59–77.

Bran, S. (1998) 'Violencia, cultura, y seguridad pública en El Salvador', *Realidad,* vol. 64 (San Salvador), pp. 325–35.

Brazilian Constitution (1988*) Constituição da república federativa do Brasil: de 5 outubro de 1988* (3rd edition) (São Paulo: Editora Atlas).

Briones, C. (1991) 'La probreza urbana en El Salvador: Características y diferencias de los hogares pobres, 1988–1990' (San Salvador: IIES–UCA), unpublished paper.

Briscoe, J. (1984) 'Water Supply and Health in Developing Countries: Selective Primary Health Care Revisited', *American Journal of Public Health,* vol. 74, pp. 1009–13.

Brodwin, P. (1996) *Medicine and Morality in Haiti: the Contest for Healing Power* (Cambridge: Cambridge University Press).

Bulmer-Thomas, V. (ed.) (1996) *The New Economic Model in Latin America and its Impact on Income Distribution and Poverty* (London: Macmillan/ Institute of Latin American Studies).

Bunge, A. (1917) *El seguro nacional* (Buenos Aires: Ediciones Siglo).

Buse, K. and Gwin, C. (1998) 'The World Bank and Global Cooperation in Health: The Case of Bangladesh', *The Lancet,* vol. 351, pp. 665–8.

Cagan, B. and Cagan, S. (1991) *This Promised Land. El Salvador. The Refugee Community of Colomancagua and their Return to Morazan* (New Brunswick: Rutgers University Press).

Caldas, M.P. and Wood Jr., T. (1997) '"For the English to See": The Importation of Managerial Technology in Late 20th-Century Brazil', *Organization*, vol. 4, no. 4, pp. 517–34

Carneiro, J.T.M. (1991) 'Proyecto de fortalecimiento de los sectores sociales. Eficiencia de personal. Informe preliminar', unpublished report to the World Bank (San Salvador).

Cassels, A. (1995) 'Health Sector Reform: Key Issues in Less Developed Countries', *Journal of International Development,* vol. 7, no. 3.

Caviedes, R.. (1996) 'El sistema privado de salud en Chile (ISAPRES)', in AGAFP (ed.), *II Congreso Iberoamericano de Sistemas de Pensiones* (Santiago: Asociación Gremial de Administradoras de Fondos de Pensiones), pp. 165–92.

CEPAL (1987) *La industria farmacéutica: desarrollo histórico y posibilidades futuras. Argentina, Brasil y México* (Santiago:CEPAL).

CEPAL (1993) *Panorama social de América Latina: 1993* (Santiago: CEPAL).

Chen, L.C. (1988) 'Ten Years after Alma Ata: Balancing Different Primary Health Care Strategies', *Tropical and Geographical Medicine*, vol. 40, pp. 522–9.

Chernichovsky, D. (1995) 'Health System Reform in Industrialized Democracies: An Emerging Paradigm', *Milbank Quarterly*, vol. 73, pp. 339–72.

CIEDESS (1994) *Modernización de la seguridad social en Chile 1980–1993: Resultados y tendencias* (Santiago).

CISS (1998) *Extensión del diagnóstico basal del PAC* (Cuernavaca, Mexico: INSP).

Cole, K. (1998) *Cuba. From Revolution to Development* (London: Cassell).

Collins, C. (1995) 'Decentralization', in K. Janovsky (ed.), *Health Policy and Systems Development* (Geneva: WHO), chapter 10, pp. 161–78.

Collins, C. and Green, A. (1994) 'Decentralization and Health Care: Some Negative Implications in Developing Countries', *International Journal of Health Services*, vol. 23, no. 3.

Conyers, D. (1983) 'Decentralization. The Territorial Dimension of the State', *Public Administration and Development*, vol. 3, pp. 97–109.

COPAZ (1993) 'Censo nacional de lisiados y discapacitados a consecuencia del conflicto armado en El Salvador. Informe de resultados generales' (San Salvador), unpublished report.

Cruz, A. (1999) 'Sólo siete estados tienen cobertura sanitaria al ciento por ciento: OPS', *La Jornada*, April 7, p. 45.

Cruz, J.M. (1998) 'Agresión, victimización y armas en los centros educativos de San Salvador', *Realidad*, vol. 64 (San Salvador), pp. 337–55.

Da Matta, R. (1990) *Carnavais, malandros e heroís: para uma sociologia do dilema Brasileiro*, 5th edition (Rio de Janeiro: Guanabara).

Da Matta, R. (1991a) *A casa e a rua*, 4th edition (Rio de Janeiro: Guanabara).

Da Matta, R. (1991b) *O que faz o Brasil?*, 5th edition (Rio de Janeiro: Rocco).

Danielson, R. (1979) *Cuban Medicine* (New Brunswick: Transaction Books).

De Carvalho, G.I. and Santos, L. (1992*) Sistema único de saúde: comentários à Lei Orgânica da Saúde* (Leis 8.080/90 and 8.142/90) (São Paulo: Editora Hucitec).

De Kadt, E. (1994) 'Getting and Using Knowledge about the Poor: With Latin American Case Material', *IDS Bulletin*, vol. 25, no. 2.

Deininger, K. and Squire, L. (1996) *Measuring Income Inequality: A New Data Base* (Washington, DC: World Bank).

Departamento de Planificación (1997) *Financiamento de la salud* (Havana: MINSAP).

Desjarlais, R., Eisenberg, L., Good, B. and Kleinman, A. (1995) *World Mental Health: Problems and Priorities in Low-Income Countries* (New York: Oxford University Press).

Dirección General de Estadística e Informática, Secretaría de Salud, México (1997) 'Información básica sobre recursos y servicios del Sistema Nacional de Salud', *Salud Pública de México*, vol. 39, no. 6, p. 590.

Dirección General de Estadística e Informática, Secretaría de Salud, México (1998) *Principales resultados de la estadística sobre mortalidad en México*, vol. 40, no. 6, pp. 515–23.

Dominguez, J. and Lowenthal, A. (eds.) (1996) *Constructing Democratic Governance: Latin America and the Caribbean in the 1990s* (Baltimore: Johns Hopkins University Press).

Duarte, D. (1995) 'Asignación de recursos per cápita en la atención primaria', *Cuadernos de Economía*, vol. 32, no. 95, pp. 117–24.

Dunkerley, J. (1982) *The Long War: Dictatorship and Revolution in El Salvador* (London: Junction Books).

Durán, L. (1990) 'La calidad de la consulta prescriptiva en atención primaria', *Salud Pública de México*, vol. 32, no. 2, pp. 181–91.

Eckstein, S. (1997) 'The Limits of Socialism in a Capitalist World Economy', in M.A. Centeno and M. Font (eds.), *Toward a New Cuba?: Legacies of a Revolution* (Boulder: Lynne Rienner).

Economist Intelligence Unit (1998) 'Profile — State and Private Healthcare Coverage in Chile', *EIU Healthcare International* (2nd quarter), pp. 37–53.

Editorial (1981) 'Un proceso de mediación para El Salvador', *Estudios Centroamericanos*, vol. 36 (San Salvador), pp. 3–16.

Editorial (1998) 'Firme y unánime rechazo a la privatización del IMSS', *Epoca*, vol. 1, no. 15 (Mexico). (In addition to the Editorial, the entire issue is devoted to expressing opposition to the Reform of IMSS).

Eisenstadt, S.N. and Roniger, L. (1984) *Patrons, Clients and Friends: Interpersonal Relations and the Structure of Trust in Society* (Cambridge: Cambridge University Press).

Engs, E., Briscoe, J. and Cunningham, A. (1990) 'Participation Effect from Water Projects on EPI', *Social Science and Medicine*, vol. 30, pp. 1349–58.

Enthoven, A. (1988) *Theory and Practice of Managed Competition in Health Care Finance* (Amsterdam: North Holland).

Estudios Centroamericanos (1992) 'Documento especial Acuerdo de Paz', *Estudios Centroamericanos*, vol. 47 (San Salvador), pp. 103–51.

Faoro, R. (1991*) Os donos do poder: formação do patronato político brasileiro*, 9th edition (São Paulo: Globo).

Feinsilver, J. (1993) *Healing the Masses: Cuban Health Politics at Home and Abroad* (San Fransisco: University of California Press).

FESAL–93 (1994) *National Family Health Survey* (San Salvador: USAID).

Fitzpatrick, R. and Hopkins, A. (1983) 'Problems in the Conceptual Framework of Patient Satisfaction Research: An Empirical Exploration', *Sociology of Health and Illness*, vol. 5, no. 3, pp. 297–311.

Flynn, P. (1993) 'Brazil: Conflict or Conciliation?', *Conflict Studies*, no. 265.

French, H. (1993) 'Cuba's Ill Encroach on Health', *The New York Times*, 16 July 1993, p. A3.

Frenk, J. (1993) 'The New Public Health', *Annual Review of Public Health*, vol. 14, pp. 469–89.

Frenk, J. (1994) 'Dimensions of Health System Reform', *Health Policy*, vol. 27, pp. 19–34.

Frenk, J. (1995) 'Comprehensive Policy Analysis for Health System Reform, *Health Policy*, vol. 32, pp. 257–77.

Frenk, J. (1998a) 'Chiapas: las desigualdades internas', *La Jornada*, 26 January, p. 7.

Frenk, J. (1998b) '20 años de salud en México', *Nexos*, January, pp. 85–91.

Frenk, J., Bobadilla, J.L. and Lozano, R. (1996) 'The Epidemiologic Transition in Latin America', in I.M. Timaeus, J. Chackiel and L. Ruzicka (eds.), *Adult Mortality in Latin America* (Oxford, New York: Clarendon Press), pp. 123–39.

Frenk, J., González-Block, M.A. and Lozano, R. (1998) 'Seis tesis equivocadas sobre las políticas de salud en el combate a la pobreza', *Este País*, no. 84, pp. 28–36.

Frenk, J., Lozano, R., González-Block, M.A. et al. (1994) *Health and the Economy: Proposals for Progress in the Mexican Health System. Overview* (México City: Fundación Mexicana para la Salud).

Fuenzalida, A. (1995) 'El nuevo modelo de financiamiento del nivel primario de atención de salud municipal: pago per cápita', *Cuadernos de Economía,* vol. 32, no. 95, pp. 125–8.

Fuenzalida-Puelma, H.L. and Scholle-Connor, S. (eds.) (1989) *The Right to Health in the Americas: A Comparative Constitutional Study* (Washington, DC: Pan American Health Organisation).

Garfield, R. (1989) *Health and Revolution. The Nicaraguan Experience* (Oxford: Oxford University Press).

Garfield, R. and Santana, S. (1997) 'The Impact of the Economic Crisis and the US Embargo on Health in Cuba', *American Journal of Public Health,* vol. 87, no. 1, pp. 15–20.

Garst, R. and Barry, T. (1990) *Feeding the Crisis. US Food Aid and Farm Policy in Central America* (Lincoln, NE: University of Nebraska Press).

Garuffi, M. (1939) 'El mutualismo en la República Argentina', PhD thesis, Faculty of Economics, National University of Buenos Aires.

Gay, R. (1990) 'Community Organization and Clientelist Politics in Contemporary Brazil: A Case Study from Rio de Janeiro', *International Journal of Urban and Regional Research,* vol. 14, no. 4, pp. 648–66.

Gerassi, J. (1963) *The Great Fear in Latin America* (New York: Collier).

Gereffi, G. (1983) *The Pharmaceutical Industry and Dependency in the Third World* (Princeton: Princeton University Press).

Gershberg, A.I. (1998) *Decentralization and Recentralization: Lessons from the Social Sectors in Mexico and Nicaragua* (Washington, DC: Social Programs Division, Region II, Inter-American Development Bank).

Gertler, P. et al. (1989) 'Are User Fees Regressive? The Welfare Implications of Charging for Medical Care in Peru', in PAHO, *Health Economics. Latin American Perspectives* (Washington, DC).

Giedion, U. and Wullner, A. (1996) *La unidad de pago por capacitación y el equilibrio financiero del sistema de salud* (Bogotá: Fedesarrollo Editorial Guadalupe).

Gilson, L., Russel, S. and Buse, K. (1995) 'The Political Economy of User Fees with Targeting: Developing Equitable Health Financing Policy', *Journal of International Development,* vol. 7, no. 3.

Glassman, A. et al. (1999) 'Applying Political Analysis to Understand Reform: The Case of the Dominican Republic', *Health Policy and Planning,* vol. 14, no. 2.

González-Block, M.A. (1994) 'Health Care Access Policy and Service Utilization. The Case of Prenatal Care and Child Delivery in Mexico', *Health Policy and Planning,* vol. 9, 204–12.

González-Block, M.A. et al. (1989) 'Health Services Decentralization in Mexico: Formulation, Implementation, and Results of Policy, *Health Policy and Planning*, vol. 4, no. 4, pp. 301–15.

González García, G. and Tobar, F. (1997) *Más salud por el mismo dinero. La reforma del sistema de salud en Argentina* (Buenos Aires: Ediciones Isalud).

González García, G. et al. (1987) *El gasto en salud y en medicamentos* (Buenos Aires: Centro de Estudios de Estado y Sociedad).

Govindaraj, R., Murray, C.J.L. and Chellaraj, G. (1994) 'Health Expenditures in Latin America', paper prepared for the Technical Department for Latin and the Caribbean (Washington, DC: World Bank)

Grindle, M. (1996) *Challenging the State: Crisis and Innovation in Latin America and Africa* (Cambridge: Cambridge University Press).

Grindle, M. and Thomas, J. (eds.) (1991) *Public Choices and Policy Change: The Political Economy of Reform in the Developing World* (Baltimore: Johns Hopkins University Press).

Grupo de Reforma del Sector Salud (1995) *Documento guía para la reforma del sector salud en El Salvador* (*borrador para discusión*) (San Salvador: Ministerio de Salud Pública y Asistencia Social).

Harvard University School of Public Health (1996) *La reforma de salud en Colombia y el plan maestro de implementación*, Informe Final, República de Colombia, Ministerio de Salud, Programa Universidad de Harvard.

Hartlyn, J. and Morley, S. (eds.) (1996) *Latin American Political Economy: Financial Crisis and Political Change* (Boulder: Westview).

Hernández, P., Zurita, B., Ramírez, R., Alvarez, F. and Cruz, C. (1997) 'Las cuentas nacionales de salud', in J. Frenk (ed.), *Observatorio de la salud: necesidades, servicios, políticas* (Mexico City: Funsalud), pp. 119–142.

Hess, D.J. and Da Matta, R.A. (eds.) (1995) *The Brazilian Puzzle: Culture on the Borderlands of the Western World* (New York: Columbia University Press).

Hill, M. (ed.) (1993) *New Agendas in the Study of the Policy Process* (Hemel Hempstead: Harvester Wheatsheaf).

Hirschman, A.O. (1970) *Exit, Voice and Loyalty: Responses to Decline in Firms, Organizations and States* (Cambridge, MA: Harvard University Press).

Hsiao, W. (1995) 'Abnormal Economics in the Health Sector', *Health Policy*, vol. 32, pp. 125–39.

Icú, H. (1998) 'El papel de la sociedad civil ante el sistema integral de atención en salud "SIAS"', paper presented at the workshop 'Health and Human Development in the New Global Economy', Galveston, Texas, October 26–28.

Instituto Mexicano del Seguro Social (1997) *Hacia el fortalecimiento y la modernización de la seguridad social* (Mexico City: IMSS).

Instituto Mexicano del Seguro Social (1998) *55 años: hacia el siglo XXI, hechos y perspectivas* (Mexico City: IMSS).

INDEC (1995) *Situación y evolución social. Síntesis no. 3* (Buenos Aires).

INDEC (1996) *Anuario estadístico de la República Argentina, 1996* (Buenos Aires).

Instituto Universitario de Opinión Pública (1998) *Delincuencia y opinión pública*, Estudios Centroamericanos, vol. 53 (San Salvador), pp. 785–802.

Inter-American Development Bank (1996) *Economic and Social Progress in Latin America. The 1996 Report* (Washington, DC: Johns Hopkins University Press for the Inter-American Development Bank).

Inter-American Development Bank (1998) 'Argentina: programa de modernización y reforma del sector salud', 13 April (http://www.iadb.org/exr/doc98/pro/uar0120.htm).

Iplance (1997) *Ranking dos municípios* (Fundação Instituto do Planejamento do Ceará, Fortaleza).

Iunes, R.S. (1994) 'Estudio: evaluación del sector privado. Proyecto análisis del sector salud de El Salvador (ANSS/ES), San Salvador, July, unpublished report.

Ivereigh, A. (1995) *Catholicism and Politics in Argentina* (London: Macmillan).

Jamison, D.T., Mosley, W.H., Measham, A.R. and Bobadilla, J.L. (eds.) (1993) *Disease Control Priorities in Developing Countries* (New York: Oxford University Press for the World Bank).

Jané Camacho, E. (1999) 'Sistemas de salud y desarrollo. Un análisis de políticas de salud para la orientación de las acciones de cooperación al desarrollo', unpublished paper.

Jaramillo, I. (1997) *El futuro de la salud en Colombia. La puesta en marcha de la ley 100*, FESCOL, Fundacíon FES, Fundacíon Restrepo Barco, Fundacíon Corona, 3rd Edition (Bogotá: Editorial Tercer Mundo).

Jaramillo, I. Olano, G. and Yepes, F. (1998) *La ley 100. Dos años de implementacíon*, ASSALUD, FESCOL, Fundacíon Corona, Fundacíon FES, GTZ, Informes Técnicos no. 2 (Bogotá: Editorial Guadalupe).

Justo, M. (1998) 'Profile-Changing Political Gears in Argentina's Healthcare System', *EIU Healthcare International*, 2nd Quarter.

Karl, T. (1996) '¿Cuánta democracia acepta la desigualdad?', *Este País*, December, pp. 46–50.

Katz, J. and Muñoz, A. (1988) *Organización del sector salud: puja distributiva y equidad* (Buenos Aires: Centro Editor de América Latina).

Kifmann, M. (1998) 'Private Insurance in Chile: Basic or Complementary Insurance for Outpatient Services?', *International Social Security Review*, vol. 51(1/98), pp. 137–52.

Kirkpatrick, A.F. (1996) 'Role of the USA in Shortage of Food and Medicine in Cuba', *The Lancet*, vol. 348, pp. 1489–91.

Knaul, F., Parker, S. and Ramírez, R. (1997) 'El prepago por servicios médicos privados en México: determinantes socio-económicos y cambios a través del tiempo', in J. Frenk (ed.), *Observatorio de la salud: necesidades, servicios, políticas* (Mexico City: Funsalud), pp. 195–213.

Kutzin, J. (1995) *Experience with Organizational and Financing Reform of the Health Sector* (Geneva: WHO, Division of Analysis, Research and Assessment. WHO/ARA/CC/97.5).

La Forgia, G. (1989) 'User Fees, Quality of Care and the Poor: Lessons from the Dominican Republic' (Washington: Inter-American Foundation).

Lara, A., Gómez-Dantés, O., Urdapilleta, O. and Bravo M.L. (1997) 'Gasto federal en salud en población no asegurada: México 1980–1995', *Salud Pública de México,* vol. 39, pp. 102–9.

Lara, T., García Ramirios, C. and de Calderón, S.E. (1994). *Rescate de la autogestión comunitaria en la solución de sus problemas de salud en las zonas conflictivas (1981–1991)* (San Salvador: DANIDA).

Larrañaga, I. (1997a) *Eficiencia y equidad en el sistema de salud chileno*, Serie Finaciamiento al Desarrollo, no. 49 (Santiago de Chile: CEPAL).

Larrañaga, O. (1997b) 'Reforms of the Health Sector in Chile', mimeo (Santiago: Department of Economics, University of Chile).

Laure, J. (1993) *El Salvador 1954–1991. Poder de compra de los salarios mínimos, antes y durante la guerra civil,* Colección Documentos Técnicos, no. 24 (Guatemala: Instituto de Nutrición de Centro América y Panamá).

Leal, V.N. (1975) *Coronelismo, enxada e voto: o município e o regime representativo no Brasil* (São Paulo: Alfa-Omega).

Lenz, R. (1995) 'Pago asociado a diagnóstico: breve reseña', *Cuadernos de Economía,* vol. 32, no. 95, pp. 105–12.

Lipsky, M. (1980) *Street Level Bureaucracy* (New York: Macmillan).

Lloyd-Sherlock, P. (1997) 'Policy, Distribution and Poverty in Argentina since Redemocratization', *Latin American Perspectives,* vol. 24, no. 6.

Lloyd-Sherlock, P. (2000) 'Failing the Needy: Public Social Spending in Latin America', *Journal of International Development,* no. 12.

Londoño, J.L. (1995a) 'La estructuración social hacia el nuevo siglo y el rol del Estado', paper prepared for the Technical Department for Latin and the Caribbean, World Bank, Washington, DC.

Londoño, J.L. (1995b) 'Poverty, Inequality and Democracy in Latin America', paper presented at the First Annual World Bank Conference on Development Economics in Latin America, Rio de Janeiro.

Londoño, J.L. and Moser, C. (1996) 'Violencia urbana en América Latina', paper presented at the Second Annual World Bank Conference on Development Economics in Latin America, Bogotá.

Lundgren R.I. and R. Lang. (1989) '"There is no Sea, only Fish": Effects of the United States' Policy on the Health of the Displaced in El Salvador', *Social Science and Medicine,* vol. 28, pp. 697–706.

Mackintosh, M. (1992) 'Questioning the State', in M. Wuyts, M. Mackintosh and T. Hewitt (eds.), *Development Policy and Public Action* (Oxford: Oxford University Press in Association with the Open University).

Madrid, I., Velázquez, G. and Fefer, E. (1998) *Pharmaceuticals and Health Sector Reform in the Americas: An Economic Perspective* (Washington: Pan American Health Organization).

Manrique, A. and Marín, F. (1987) *Ley 12. Decentralizacíon administrativa y fiscal,* Serie: Reforma Política, no. 3 (FESCOL, Procomún, Bogotá, May).

Marcel, M. and Arenas, A. (1992) 'Social Security Reform in Chile', Occasional Paper no. 5. (Washington, DC: Inter-American Development Bank).

Martín-Baró, I. (1981) 'La guerra civil en El Salvador', *Estudios Centroamericanos,* vol. 36 (San Salvador), pp. 17–32.

McClintock, M. (1985) *The American Connection: State Terror and Popular Resistance in El Salvador* (London: Zed Books).

MacDonald, J.J. (1993) *Primary Health Care. Medicine in its Place* (London: Earthscan).

McGreevey, W.P. (1988) 'The High Costs of Health Care in Brazil', *PAHO Bulletin,* vol. 22, no. 2, pp. 145–66

McGreevey, W. (1990) *Social Security in Latin America: Issues and Options for the World Bank* (Washington, DC: World Bank).

Medeiros, R.L.R. (1997) *Práticas políticas no interior Cearense: as eleições municipais do 1996 em Caridade,* Masters dissertation, Department of Sociology, Federal University of Ceará, Fortaleza.

Medina, A. (1997) 'La transicíon del sistema', in H. Sánchez Luz and F. Yepes (eds.), *La ley 100. Dos años de implementacíon,* ASSALUD, FESCOL, Fundacíon Corona, Fundacíon FES, GTZ. Informes Técnicos no.1 (Bogotá: Editorial Guadalupe).

Mensa, J. (1946) 'Algunas consideraciones sobre legislación mutual', *Crónica Mensual de la Secretaría de Trabajo y Previsión* (Buenos Aires, January 1946).

Mesa-Lago, C. (1992) *Health Care for the Poor in Latin America and the Caribbean* (Washington: Pan American Health Organisation).

Mesa-Lago, C. (1997) 'Social Welfare Reform in the Context of Economic-Political Liberalization: Latin American Cases', *World Development,* vol. 25, no. 4, pp. 497–517.

Mideplan (1990) *Programas sociales: su impacto en los hogares chilenos* (Santiago: Ministerio de Planificación y Cooperación).

Mideplan (1991) 'Los sistemas previsionales de salud. Cobertura y perfil de los beneficiarios', *Documentos Sociales* (Santiago: Ministerio de Planificación y Cooperación).

Mideplan (1996) *Balance de seis años de las políticas sociales 1990–1996* (Santiago: Ministerio de Planificación y Cooperación).

Mills, A. (1983) 'Economic Aspects of Health Insurance', in K. Lee and A. Mills (eds.), *The Economics of Healthcare in Developing Countries* (Oxford: Oxford University Press).

Mills, A. (1998a) 'To Contract or not to Contract? Issues for Low and Middle Income Countries', *Health Policy and Planning,* vol. 13, pp. 32–40.

Mills, A. (1998b) 'Health Care Reforms in Developing Countries', *Informing and Reforming,* no. 5, pp. 2–5.

Ministerio de Planeación. Unidad de Investigaciones Muestrales (1990) *Encuesta de hogares de propósitos multiples. Total país urbano* (San Salvador).

Ministerio de Salud (1994) *La carga de la enfermedad* (Bogotá).

Ministerio de Salud (1998a) 'Estadísticas', web site, Ministerio de Salud: www.minsal.cl.

Ministerio de Salud (1998b) 'Modernización del sector público de salud', web site, Ministerio de Salud: www.minsal.cl.

Ministerio de Salud Pública y Asistencia Social (1994) *Plan Nacional de Salud (1994–1999). Pérfil* (San Salvador).

MINSAP (1997) *Políticas de salud actual* (Havana: MINSAP).

Miranda, E. (1989) 'Desarrollo y perspectivas del sistema de ISAPRES', *Documento Serie Investigación*, no. 94 (Santiago: Departamento de Economía, Universidad de Chile).

Miranda, E. (ed.) (1994) *La salud en Chile: Evolución y perspectivas* (Santiago: Centro de Estudios Públicos).

Miranda, E., Scarpaci, J.L. and Irarrázaval I. (1995) 'A Decade of HMOs in Chile: Market Behaviour, Consumer Choice and the State', *Health and Place*, vol. 1, no. 1, pp. 51–9.

Montgomery, T.S. (1995) *Revolution in El Salvador. From Civil Strife to Civil Peace* (Boulder: Westview Press).

Mooney, G. (1987) 'What does Equity in Health Mean?', *World Statistics Quarterly*, no. 40.

Mora, José Obdulio (1982) *Situación nutricional de la población colombiana en1977–80. Volúmen I: Resultados antropométricos y de laboratorio. Comparación con 1965–66*, Estudio Nacional de Salud. Ministerio de Salud. Instituto Nacional de Salud. Asociación Colombiana de Facultades de Medicina (Bogotá, July).

Morel, A. (1991) *Refugiados salvadoreños en Nicaragua* (Managua: ACRES).

Morley, S. (1995) *Poverty and Inequality in Latin America. The Impact of Adjustment and Recovery in the 1980s* (Baltimore: Johns Hopkins University Press).

Morrison, A. and Orlando, M. (1997) *The Socio-Economic Impact of Domestic Violence against Women in Chile and Nicaragua* (Washington: Inter-American Development Bank).

Munck, R. (1998) 'Mutual Benefit Societies in Argentina: Workers, Nationality, Social Security and Trade Unionism', *Journal of Latin American Studies*, vol. 30, no. 3, pp. 573–90.

Murray, C. and Lozano, R. (1996) 'The Burden of Disease in Latin America', paper prepared for the Technical Department for Latin America and the Caribbean, World Bank, Washington, DC.

Musgrove, P. (1996) 'Public and Private Roles in Health: Theory and Financing Patterns', World Bank Discussion Paper No. 339 (Washington, DC: The World Bank).

Nickson, A. (1995) *Local Government in Latin America* (Boulder: Lynne Rienner).

Nigenda, G. (1997) 'The Regional Distribution of Doctors in Mexico, 1930–1990: A Policy Assessment', *Health Policy,* vol. 39, no. 2.

North, D.C. (1990) *Institutions and Institutional Development* (Cambridge: Cambridge University Press).

Oakes, M.G. (1998) 'Emotional Reactions to the Trauma of War: A Field Study in Rural El Salvador', doctoral dissertation, School of Social Work, University of Texas, Austin.

Olubo, S.O. (1994) 'The Medical Profession and Health Policy in Nigeria', *Studies in Third World Development,* vol. 55, pp. 3–19.

OPS (1984) *Participación de la comunidad en la salud y el desarrollo de las Américas,* Publicación Científica, no. 473 (Washington, DC: Pan American Health Organisation).

Organisation for Economic Cooperation and Development (1992) *The Reform of Health Care: A Comparative Analysis of Seven OECD Countries,* Health Policy Studies No. 2 (Paris: OECD).

Oxley, H. and MacFarlan, M. (1994*) Health Care Reform. Controlling Spending and Increasing Efficiency,* Economics Department Working Paper 149 (Paris: OECD).

Oyarzo, C. (1994) 'La mezcla público-privada. Una reforma pendiente en el sector salud', in E. Miranda (ed.), *La Salud en Chile: Evolución y Perspectivas* (Santiago: Centro de Estudios Públicos).

Oyarzo, C. and Galleguillos, S. (1995) 'Reforma del sistema de salud chileno: marco conceptual de la propuesta del Fondo Nacional de Salud', *Cuadernos de Economía,* vol. 32, no. 95, pp. 29–46.

Palmeira, M. (1993) 'Política, facção e compromiso – alguns significados do voto', *IV Encontro de Ciências Sociais no Nordeste,* Salvador, December.

PAMSP (c.1995) *Modernización del sector público de El Salvador* (San Salvador).

Pan American Health Organisation (1994) *Health Conditions in the Americas* (Washington, DC: PAHO).

Pan American Health Organisation (1995a) *Health Conditions in the Americas,* Scientific Publication no. 549 (Washington, DC: PAHO).

Pan American Health Organisation (1995b) 'Country Health Profiles. Argentina', http://www.paho.org/english/argentin.htm.

Pan American Health Organisation (1996) *Resumen ejecutivo: ciclo de conferencias sobre la economía Cubana* (Havana).

Pan American Health Organisation (1997) *Cooperation of the Pan American Health Organisation in Health Sector Reform Processes.* (Washington, DC: PAHO).

Pan American Health Organisation (1998) *Health in the Americas* (Washington, DC: PAHO).

Pan American Health Organisation (PAHO) (1999) *Epidemiological Bulletin,* vol. 20, no. 1 (March).

Pearce, J. (1982) *Under the Eagle. US Intervention in Central America and the Caribbean* (London: Latin America Bureau).

PNUD (1994) *La hora de la paz. Desarrollo humano y salud mental. Experiencias en Centroamérica* (El Salvador).

Portillo, N. (1998) 'Armas de fuego: ¿una respuesta a la inseguridad ciudadana? Su impacto y prevalencia en la morbilidad del AMSS', *Realidad,* vol. 64 (San Salvador), pp. 357–80.

Pressman, J. and Wildavsky, A. (1973) *Implementation: How Great Hopes in Washington are Dashed in Oakland* (Berkeley: University of California Press).

PRISMA (1995) *El Salvador: Dinámica de la degradación ambiental* (San Salvador: PRISMA).

Puyana, A. (1993) 'The Campaign against Absolute Poverty in Colombia: An Evaluation of Liberal Social Policy', in C. Abel and C. Lewis (eds.), *Welfare, Poverty and Development in Latin America* (Basingstoke: Macmillan).

Quevedo, Emilio (1990) 'Análisis sociohistórico', in Francisco J. Yepes (director) *La Salud en Colombia*, Estudio Sectorial de Salud, Ministerio de Salud, Departamento Nacional de Planeación (Bogotá: Editorial Presencia).

Ramírez Martínez, J.D. (1998) 'Health Care Reform and Civil Society in Post-Conflict Conditions. El Salvador', paper presented at the workshop 'Health and Human Development in the New Global Economy', Galveston, Texas, October 26–28.

Recalde, H. (1991) *Beneficencia, asistencialismo estatal y previsión social/1* (Buenos Aires: Centro Editor de América Latina).

Reich, M. (1995) 'The Politics of Health Sector Reform in Developing Countries: Three Cases of Pharmaceutical Policy', in Peter Berman

P. (ed.), *Health Sector Reform in Developing Countries* (Boston: Harvard School of Public Health).

Rodrigues, J. (1989) 'What is Happening to Hospital Utilization in Brazil?', *Health Policy and Planning,* vol. 4, pp. 354–9.

Rodríguez, L. (1995) 'Prestaciones complejas', *Cuadernos de Economía,* vol. 32, no. 95, pp. 113–6.

Roemer, M.I. (1991) *National Health Systems of the World, Vol. 1: The Countries* (New York: Oxford University Press).

Rogers, P. (1996) 'Implementation of Health Care in Brazil', in *Policymaking in a Redemocratized Brazil,* Research Report No. 119 (Austin: University of Texas).

Rojas Ochoa, F. and López Pardo, C.M. (1997) 'Economy, Politics, and Health Status in Cuba', *International Journal of Health Services,* vol. 27, no. 4, pp. 791–807.

Rosenberg, T. (1999) 'What did you do in the War, Mama?', *New York Times Magazine,* Feb. 7, pp. 48ff.

Ruiz, A., Askin, P.W. and Gibb, D.C. (1978) *Health Sector Assessment. El Salvador* (Washington DC: USAID).

Ruiz, Hugo and Torres, Jorge (1990) *Seguridad social. Volumen I: Características de la población,* Ministerio de Salud. Instituto de Seguros Sociales. Instituto Nacional de Salud. Bogotá (July).

Sánchez Luz, H. and Yepes, F. (1998) (eds.) *La ley 100. Dos años de implementacíon,* ASSALUD, FESCOL, Fundacíon Corona, Fundacíon FES, GTZ, Informes Técnicos No. 1 (Editorial Guadalupe: Bogotá).

Schmitter, P.C. (1979) 'Still the Century of Corporatism?', in P.C. Schmitter and G. Lehmbruch (eds.), *Trends toward Corporatist Intermediation* (Beverly Hills and London: SAGE Publications), pp. 7–52.

Secretaría de Salud (1994) *Encuesta Nacional de Salud II* (Mexico City: SSA).

Secretaría de Salud (1997) *Principales líneas de trabajo de la Secretaría de Salud. Síntesis* (Mexico City: Secretaría de Salud).

Secretária de Saúde, Ceará (1992) *O Ceará e a municipalização da saúde: encontro com os novos prefeitos do Ceará* (Governo do Estado do Ceará).

Shore, C. and Wright, S. (1997) 'Policy: A New Field of Anthropology', in C. Shore and S. Wright (eds.) *Anthropology of Policy* (London: Routledge), chapter 1, 3–39.

Silva, H. (September 1995) Conference Imparted at the National Association of Nurses, San Salvador (Dr Silva was a member of the Asamblea Nacional Convergencia Democrática).

Silverman, M. (1976) *The Drugging of the Americas* (Berkeley, London: University of California Press).

Starr, P. (1994) *The Logic of Health Care Reform* (New York: Whittle Books).

Stillwaggon, E. (1998) *Stunted Lives, Stagnant Economies. Poverty, Disease and Underdevelopment* (London: Rutgers University Press).

Stocker, K., Waitzkin, H. and Iriart, C. (1999) 'The Exportation of Managed Care to Latin America', *New England Journal of Medicine*, vol. 340, no. 14, pp. 1131–6.

Superintendencia de la Seguridad Social (1998) *Estadísticas de la Seguridad Social 1997* (Santiago: Superintendencia de Seguridad Social).

Tedesco, Laura (2001, forthcoming) 'The 1999 Elections in Argentina: Change in Style or Substance?', *European Review of Latin American and Caribbean Studies*, April 2001.

Teitel, S. (ed.) (1992) *Towards a New Development Strategy for Latin America: Pathways from Hirschman's Thought* (Washington, DC: Inter-American Development Bank).

Tendler, J (1997) *Good Government in the Tropics* (Baltimore: Johns Hopkins University Press).

Thorp, R. (1991) 'Introduction', in C. Abel and C. Lewis (eds.) *Latin America: Economic Imperialism and the State* (Basingstoke: Macmillan).

Trejo, C. and Jones, C. (1993) *Contra la pobreza. Por una estrategia de política social* (Mexico City: Cal y Arena).

Trumper, R. and Phillips, L. (1997) 'Give me Discipline and Give me Death: Neoliberalism and Health in Chile', *International Journal of Health Services,* vol. 27, no. 1.

Tulchin, J. and Romero, B. (eds.) (1995) *The Consolidation of Democracy in Latin America* (Boulder: Lynne Rienner Publishers).

Ugalde, A. (1985) 'Ideological Dimensions of Community Participation in Latin America Health Programs', *Social Science and Medicine*, vol. 32, pp. 41–53.

Ugalde, A. (1998) 'Un acercamiento teórico a la participación comunitaria en salud', *Carta Médica,* no. 12 (Bolivia), pp. 42–9.

Ugalde, A. and Homedes, N. (1988) 'Towards a Rural Health Corps Concept: Lessons from the Dominican Republic', *Journal of Rural Health*, vol. 4, pp. 41–58.

Ugalde, A., Homedes, N. and Rochwerger, D. (1988) *Estudio de Consulta Externa* (San José: Development Technologies Inc.).

Ugalde, A. and Zwi, A. (eds.) (1994) *Violencia política y salud en América Latina* (Mexico City: Nueva Imagen).

Ugalde, A. et al. (1996) Reconstruction *and Development of the Health Sector in El Salvador after the 1981–1992 war,* a report to the European Union in fulfilment of contract no. TS 38–CT94–03–5 (DG 12 HSMU), San Salvador.

UNICEF (1995) *Clearing the Minefields: A Step Towards Peace* (San Salvador).

Vargas, J. and Sarmiento, A. (1997*) La decentralizacíon de los servicios de salud en Colombia,* Comisíon Económica para América Latina y el Caribe, Serie Reformas de Política Pública, no. 51 (Santiago de Chile).

Velandia, F. et al. (1990) 'Financiamiento', in F. Yepes, (ed.) *La salud en Colombia. Estudio sectorial de salud,* vol. II, Ministerio de Salud, Departamento Nacional de Planeacíon (Bogotá: Editorial Presencia).

Vellozo, V.R.O. and de Souza, R.G. (1993) 'Acesso e hierarquização: um caminho (re)construído', in R.C. de A. Bodstein (ed.) *Serviços locais de saúde: construção de atores e políticas* (Rio de Janeiro: Dumará), chapter 4, 97–115.

Verdugo, J.C. (1998) 'Los riesgos de la reforma del sector salud y el papel de la sociedad civil en Guatemala. Entre una economía de guerra y una economía de mercado', paper presented at the workshop 'Health and Human Development in the New Global Economy', Galveston, Texas, October 26–28.

Veronelli, J. (1975) *Medicina, gobierno y sociedad* (Buenos Aires: Editorial El Coloquio).

Wainer, U. (1997) *Hacia una mayor equidad en la salud: el caso de las ISAPREs,* Serie Financiamiento del Desarrollo, no. 54 (Santiago de Chile: CEPAL).

Warren, K.S. (1988) 'The Evolution of Selective Primary Health Care', *Social Science and Medicine,* vol. 26, pp. 891–8.

Weyland, K. (1995) Social Movements and the State: The Politics of Health Reform in Brazil, *World Development,* vol. 23, no. 1, pp. 1699–712.

World Bank (1987) *Argentina. Population, Health, and Nutrition. Sector Review,* Report no. 6555 (Washington, DC, Oct. 26).

World Bank (1989) 'Financing Health Services in Developing Countries. An Agenda for Reform', in Pan American Health Organisation, *Health Economics. Latin American Perspectives* (Washington, DC: PAHO).

World Bank (1991) *El Salvador. Social Sector Rehabilitation Project,* Staff Appraisal Report no. 9533–ES (Washington, DC)

World Bank (1993a) *World Development Report 1993: Investing in Health* (New York: Oxford University Press for the World Bank).

World Bank (1993b) *Argentina. From Insolvency to Growth* (Washington, DC: World Bank).

World Bank (1994) *Averting the Old Age Crisis. Policies to Protect the Old and Promote Growth* (Oxford).

World Bank (1995) 'El Salvador. Health Sector Reform Project', Staff Appraisal Report, draft (Washington, DC, November 8).

World Bank (1997) *Argentina. Facing the Challenge of Health Insurance Reform* (Washington, DC).

World Health Organisation (1978) *Primary Health Care* (Geneva).

World Health Organisation (1985) 'Planning of the Finances for Health for All' (Geneva).

Yesudian, C.A.K. (1994) 'The Implementation of Health Policies in India: The Role of Physicians', *Studies in Third World Development,* vol. 55, pp. 41–56.

Yepes, F.J. (director) (1990a) *La Salud en Colombia. Estudio Sectorial de Salud,* Ministerio de Salud. Departamento Nacional de Planeación (Bogotá: Editorial Presencia), vol. 1, p. 65.

Yepes, F.J. (director) (1990b) *La Salud en Colombia. Estudio Sectorial de Salud,* Ministerio de Salud. Departamento Nacional de Planeación (Bogotá: Editorial Presencia), vol. II, p. 60.

Yepes, F.J., Sánchez, L.H. and Cantor, B. (1999) *La decentralización de salud: el caso de tres municipios colombianos,* OPS/OMS Investigaciones en Salud Pública, Documentos Técnicos.

Zuvekas, C. (1997) 'Latin America's Struggle for Equitable Economic Adjustment', *Latin American Research Review,* vol. 32, no. 2, pp. 152–69.